MY COVID DIARY

*(with a few other important topics
thrown in along the way)*

MY COVID DIARY

A PERSONAL TAKE

To remind everybody of just what we went through and how some of us rebelled.

LIZ HODGKINSON

Design, typesetting and publishing by UK Book Publishing.

www.ukbookpublishing.com

ISBN: 978-1-917329-24-8

Dedication

TO NOVAK DJOKOVIC, perhaps the greatest male tennis player of all time, who successfully and bravely refused the Covid vaccines.

Ever since the first case of what came to be called Coronavirus-19 was documented in the UK on 31ˢᵗ January 2020, I have been following the progress of the alleged pandemic, or, rather, the response to it, with ever-sinking heart.

Technically known as SARS -coV-2, or Severe Acute Respiratory Syndrome caused by a coronavirus – the same kind of virus that causes colds – its advent was followed by draconian measures such as the world had never before seen. But were the masks, lockdowns, distancing measures, school and business closures, testing, vaccines and other measures really necessary?

In this collection of essays, mostly initially published on *The Conservative Woman* website, I am arguing that they were not only completely needless and futile but caused immense harm and distress, not to mention in some cases splitting families apart beyond repair.

The main question I raise throughout this compilation is: how is it that some of us saw through to the truth very quickly, when most of the world's population didn't, and in many cases still don't? What seemed all too obvious to me, almost from the start, was apparently hidden from the majority.

I am not a scientist or a doctor and have no axe to grind, no money to make, no job or accolade to gain or lose, and no reputation to enhance or diminish either. I am a journalist and not a technical person, so this collection consists of my own experience of what I believe constitutes one of the biggest crimes against humanity since --- since when? Since ever, probably. Although terrible cruelties have been inflicted on people through wars and religion, nothing has ever gripped the entire world in such fear as Covid. And the fear wasn't even real! There was in fact nothing to fear.

Yet even in 2024, people are still testing themselves with the unreliable PCR (Polymerase Chain Reaction) test, still wearing masks, still lining up for the vaccine booster, still defending lockdown, even long after all of these measures have been discredited, initially by a few brave souls who spoke out – and often put their jobs and livelihoods on the line as a result – and gradually by ever more people as the evidence mounted up and stared them in the face.

I hope that by collecting these essays and articles into one volume, they will tell the story of how the whole debacle unfolded, written from one person's perspective. I have avoided the wilder shores of what might be termed conspiracy theories and just reported on how things have seemed to me.

The essays start in June 2021, a year and three months after the first lockdown was imposed on March 23, 2020 and six months after the first Covid vaccine was approved for use in the UK, by which time it seemed clear to me what was really going on, and that it was nothing to do with people's health and wellbeing. Just the opposite, in fact. I couldn't just stay silent, but had to speak out, and I am so grateful for *The Conservative Woman* team for being brave enough to publish these articles, at a time when no mainstream outlet would have dared to do so.

Now, four years on from the start of the Covid fearmongering, perhaps people are beginning to forget what we were made to go through, sometimes under extreme duress, so I hope this collection will remind readers of those dreadful years when just about all of life was put on hold. If we don't speak out, it could happen again. We must not allow it.

I also hope that, by reading these entries, people will come to see how ridiculous and what an utter farce the whole Covid episode was, from start to finish.

When will things get back to how they were?

GOING TO RESTAURANTS AND BARS at the moment is a miserable experience indeed. Of course I am glad that they have re-opened for indoor service, but things are far from being back to normal.

Last week I went to the DIY chain B&Q for some garden stuff wearing a completely unnecessary mask – they wouldn't let me in otherwise – and then I thought I would have a coffee in a nearby Costa. I went in and was asked to put my 'test and trace app' on the scanner. 'I don't have the app,' I said, adding: 'and I have no intention whatever of downloading it.' The staff refused to serve me and I had to go out without my coffee.

Now, I have not had Covid-19, I am perfectly fit and healthy and am not succumbing to the guilt-tripping 'Protect your loved ones with the Official NHS Covid Tracing App' thanks very much. Nor am I so paranoid or fearful that I want to know the threat level in my area – completely non-existent – or when I am near an infected person: once again a non-existent risk.

Yet you are treated as a selfish covidiot if you dare to raise a voice in protest against being tracked and traced everywhere you go. It seems as if you refuse to kowtow and download the app, you are regarded as a walking plague rat about to infect the entire world.

My next outing was not much better. I had booked a table for lunch with a friend at a country pub where we have met many times. At the door a waitress asked me to put my test and trace app on the scanner. I gave her my spiel: 'I don't have the app and I have no intention of downloading it.'

She looked doubtful, or as doubtful as one can look wearing a ridiculous mask (which staff are forced to do) and called the manager. After consulting the reservations list he was satisfied that he had all my contact details, and let me in. While waiting for my friend, who was stuck in traffic, I asked if they had any bread or olives I could nibble in the meantime. 'No, sorry,' she mumbled through her mask and handed me the menu.

It was a vastly reduced list with not many options. My friend arrived. She deliberately sticks to a dumbphone where downloading apps is impossible, but because I was already seated and the other diners had not fallen dead around me, they let her in.

On another occasion I was meeting some friends for dinner at a favourite restaurant in Oxford. We were not allowed in without our masks, which we had to wear from the door to our table, and again if we wanted to go to the loo.

It's the same story in every pub and reataurant at the moment. I'm not blaming the owners or managers. They are understandably terrified of somebody alerting the authorities if they don't adhere to these ridiculous rules, and of being shut down. But the result is that all social activity currently feels as if it is taking place under siege conditions. Every element of enjoyment has been sucked out thanks to the relentless policing.

I have to speak to my hairdresser through a mask and she is wearing not only a mask but also a visor, ensuring that there can be no meaningful conversation between us. I am not allowed to put my coat in the cloakroom but have to take it to a nearby chair. The magazines that used to be there to flip through have all been removed, and they no longer serve coffee. Once again I am not blaming the hair salons; they are too terrified of being shut down if they deviate one inch from these daft rules. I did ask my hairdresser whether anybody with Covid or who had tested positive had come into the salon. She said, 'No, not one.'

My nail technician not only wears a mask but has a Perspex screen separating her from her clients. She dares not deviate from the rules because she has nasty neighbours who are only too ready and willing to snitch on her. We used to chat but because we are both wearing masks and distancing, I can't make out what she is saying, especially as she is Croatian.

The worst aspect of all this is how many supposedly intelligent people are willing to go along with these hastily imposed and ill-thought -out restrictions. On Facebook the other day somebody posted a photo of a group of people on a train WITHOUT MASKS, as if this was the most terrible, selfish thing anybody could do. A friend took a photo of her husband and daughter on a tube train and posted it on Facebook. Neither was wearing a mask and the first question asked was: 'Why are they not wearing masks?'

No food or drink is currently served on the railways and so many seats are out of action that when you travel, it feels as though you are on a ghost train. Nothing seems real any more. It's as if we are living in a science-fiction movie come to life.

And then, just when we thought things were at last about to ease up, we are being warned that 'freedom day' is likely to be delayed for two to four weeks. I'm not holding my breath – well I am, because I can't breathe through these masks – but I will not be a bit surprised if, when we get to the middle of July, suddenly another new variant is announced, and our lives continue to be on hold.

The weak and feeble churches

IN 1797 SAMUEL TAYLOR COLERIDGE wrote these lines:

> *O sweeter than the marriage feast*
> *Tis sweeter far to me*
> *To walk together to the kirk*
> *In a goodly company.*

This verse, which also became a popular hymn, is taken from that strange gothic masterpiece, *The Rime of the Ancient Mariner.* It expresses a profound truth, that for hundreds of years people have walked together to the kirk, the church, the synagogue, the temple, the mosque, the meeting house, to worship their God in a goodly company.

Until now, when, if they walk to church at all, it is in an isolated household 'bubble.' The services when they get there are hedged about with so many rules on numbers, singing, social distancing and mask-wearing that large numbers of former churchgoers have decided it is hardly worth bothering to go at all. Whatever going to church once meant – and the spirit of community was at the heart of it – has been lost, perhaps for ever.

Oxford, where I live, has many magnificent churches and cathedrals, some dating back to the eleventh century and although most are now open, up to a point, they are nowhere near to what they were before lockdown. This is the latest notice from Christchurch, where once visitors flocked from all over the world to hear evensong:

Please note that the Cathedral has taken many steps to ensure it is COVID secure, including the introduction of ticketing for many services. You must have a ticket to attend this event (evensong). Unfortunately we will not be able to accommodate those who arrive without a ticket. Please help keep the Cathedral safe for all by following the instructions of Cathedral staff, remaining in your household group and leaving promptly after the service has finished. Do not attend if you are showing symptoms of COVID-19 or are awaiting the result of a test for COVID-19.

Whilst we will endeavour to make sure this event runs we must comply with all local, national and church guidelines, as such we may have to cancel or alter this event at short notice.

This is hardly a joyous welcome to all, is it?

Indeed, church services as we once knew them may never come back. The Church of England's website says that many congregations will continue to stream services and meet online, even if and when all restrictions end. The 'goodly company' of old will decline into a few stragglers.

Other faiths may have got so used to holding online services that they may never find the resolve to organize and hold large gatherings again. Online will, if we are not careful, become a way of life and everything will be virtual, not real.

In the past, religions prevailed against often impossible odds and faith moved mountains. Early Christians risked being burned at the stake or thrown to the lions. Yet not even the most terrible persecutions would shake their faith, and Christianity became the world's most successful religion, founded on the blood of its martyrs.

They would certainly not have let a little thing like a virus from which more than 99 per cent of people recover put them off meeting to worship their God.

In Soviet Russia, Christians were persecuted and many places of worship were destroyed. Did religion die away? It did not. People met secretly in each other's homes, often putting themselves in great danger. Since the collapse of the Soviet Union churches are full again, thanks to the brave believers who kept the faith alive.

But here, at a time when the comfort of religion is needed more than ever, where are the religious leaders telling us to take no notice of lockdowns and distancing and instead, enjoining us to hold hands, come close, worship in goodly numbers and fight the good fight with all our might?

They are nowhere. They are in retreat. Instead of showing the courage of their founding fathers, they have become craven, fearful and timid. Their swords remain sleeping in their hands.

Throughout the ages, rites of passage such as weddings, funerals and baptisms have been celebrated or marked publicly with a religious service. In more recent times, humanist services have come in for non-believers, but the sentiment is the same: people are gathering to commemorate an important life event with each other. Now, this is not happening and such events are going unmarked.

Just recently, two long-time friends of mine got married. They had hoped for a blessing in Canterbury Cathedral, but this was delayed and delayed until in the end they felt they couldn't wait any longer. They married in a register office with just two witnesses and no celebration, no fuss, no cake, nothing to make the day special in any way. Some people have said that they welcome smaller weddings. Maybe they do, but that's not the point. The choice has been taken away.

This scenario reached its nadir with the pathetic funeral of the Duke of Edinburgh. After 73 years of service to the sovereign and the state, and at nearly a hundred years of age, he, if anybody should have been given a full state funeral. Instead, selected members of the royal family shuffled along in black crow-like masks, and the poor old Queen had to sit on her own with no member of her family nearby. The only singing came from six socially-distanced members of a choir. Fashion writers raved over the elegance of the Duchess of Cambridge's outfit and not one drew attention to the fact that it was completely ruined by her black mask. Indeed, masks themselves have become a fashion statement, although on anybody apart from hospital theatre staff they look ridiculous.

Jesus himself was hardly the gentle, meek and mild saviour of popular myth. Not only did he overturn the tables of the moneylenders in the temple, he defied both the Jewish and the Roman authorities – and paid the ultimate price – to establish the new world order. If all the faiths banded together and as one, declared that they would ignore the Covid regulations that threaten to destroy them, they would form a mighty army which could, as in the past, move mountains.

Covid, the celebrity disease of our time?

DOES ANYBODY ELSE HAVE THE sneaking suspicion that one reason so many people want to keep Covid going is that it has become the celebrity disease of our time?

As Chief Medical Officer Chris Whitty announces that we won't be back to normal until at least next spring – the date for 'normal' keeps being put back and back – it could be that Covid has acquired such cult status that we might be lost without it. Where would our 'heroic' doctors and nurses be if they had to treat just ordinary, prosaic diseases such as flu and pneumonia again?

Every now and again, a disease acquires a kind of glamour that is seen as carrying off the brightest and the best, the talented, sensitive souls who are cut off in their prime. In the 1980s it was Aids, talked up as the plague of our time, and in the eighteenth and nineteenth centuries it was tuberculosis, or consumption, whose literary and romantic associations continued until the invention of antibiotics.

We remember the immortal like of Keats: 'Where youth grows pale, and spectre-thin and dies', and John Keats himself became the poster boy of tuberculosis, dying from the disease at the age of 25. Much literature was inspired by tuberculosis and Charlotte Bronte, whose two sisters died from it, wrote: 'Consumption, I am aware, is a flattering malady.'

And so is Covid. As with TB, going down with symptoms puts sufferers in a more flattering light, conferring both bravery and tragedy on them. If they were ordinary people, before, they become special once they test positive for Covid.

It's almost as if we have to have an illness or infection in our midst which is a badge of honour and which conveys instant sainthood on both the sufferers and those who look after them. Princess Diana is remembered for many things, chief of which perhaps was her embracing of emaciated Aids patients when others kept their distance. And since last year, most of us have vivid pictures in our minds of front-line medical staff, all masked up and in scrubs, courageously putting their own health on the line to treat the victims of this new and apparently life-threatening complaint.

It did not take long, once Covid-19 was identified last year, for it to become a celebrity's condition. The first such, as I recall, to test positive was former Page Three girl Linda Lusardi. Aged 62 and practically forgotten, the diagnosis of Covid brought her right back into the public eye. Pictures from her glory days were plastered all over the media and her recovery was closely monitored in the tabloids where she first sprang to topless fame.

Prime Minister Boris Johnson's admission to hospital turned Covid into a superstar illness, as doctors fought bravely to save his life. After that, sports stars, television personalities and others in the public eye began announcing that they had tested positive.

11

Famous names such as Esther Rantzen stated that they were self-isolating. Would they have made these announcements if they had gone down with winter flu or a bad cold? Of course not. But Covid added a kind of lustre to their reputation. Even the most glamorous, the most feted, were not immune.

As if Covid itself was not enough, we soon had 'long Covid' which turned sufferers even more rapidly into saints and martyrs. The latest victim of long Covid to hit the public prints was Martha Hancock, estranged wife of former health secretary Matt. A huge outpouring of sympathy was extended to her as she was pictured walking her dog, looking brave and resilient as she coped valiantly with the double whammy of being dumped by her husband and battling long Covid.

Thanks to Covid, she has now become a celebrity in her own right and you can bet that she has been offered huge sums to tell her story, with special emphasis on the Covid she apparently caught from the very husband who betrayed her. Not to be outdone, TV presenter Andrew Marr stated that he had gone down with Covid after two vaccinations.

One doesn't like to be too cynical, but when television presenter Kate Garraway's husband Derek Draper went down with Covid (very serious in his case) Kate did not stay away from the limelight but appeared as a cover girl on just about every magazine and was treated to photoshoots in designer outfits as she described in tearful detail her husband's fight with the condition. One can only say that her celebrity status was heightened thereby.

The doctors who developed the Oxford AstraZeneca vaccine also became instant celebrities. Former backroom girls Professor

Sarah Gilbert and Professor Catherine Green were hailed as 'The women who saved the world' in a cover article for the Times magazine, although the adulatory headline was toned down online. Professor Gilbert, by now Dame Sarah, was also accorded a seat in the Royal Box at Wimbledon where crowds cheered Andy Murray saying that doctors and nurses should be given a big pay rise. Murray himself earned considerable brownie points for being so caring, although it was not his money that would be funding the pay rises he was recommending.

And once Covid took a firm grip, could the books, plays and poems be far behind?

No. As with Aids and tuberculosis before, the infection has already acted as inspiration to writers and no doubt before long there will be musicals and paintings about the disease. The books are already coming thick and fast, written by survivors, doctors and others.

Earlier this year, 81-year-old Ray Connolly, who was in hospital for six months with Covid, quickly wrote a play about the condition called *Devoted*, which was performed on radio. Since his recovery, Connolly has become a kind of lockdown spokesman, and says he will be 'disappointed' if compulsory mask-wearing ends on July 19th. His celebrity status has also been greatly increased by his near-death brush. Once an elderly writer somewhat past his prime, he is now right back in the public eye. Michael Rosen, who spent 48 days in intensive care, has written *Many Different Kinds of Love*, a poetic book about the illness that he says, completely changed him.

None of this is to deny that Covid can be a serious illness as indeed were Aids and TB. But is it too much to wonder if it has become a branch of showbiz with ever more people jumping onto the bandwagon?

What has happened to our gyms?

ALTHOUGH I AM HURTLING WITH indecent haste towards my ninth decade, I remain as fit and healthy as somebody 30 or 40 years younger.

When asked what my secret is, I reply: exercise. For the past 40 years I have visited the gym several times a week, doing a variety of tough classes as well as working out on the machines. I am convinced that this regime has enabled me to stay free from such age-related conditions as diabetes, high blood pressure, osteoporosis and arthritis.

It's not just me. The former Countdown host Anne Robinson, the same age as me, said in a recent interview that regular exercise was the main reason she still had the energy to host a television programme in her mid-seventies. Anne, too, is as lithe and slim as somebody decades younger. She added that she did workouts not because they were fun but because she wanted to stay fighting fit for as long as possible.

We oldie exercisers were able to keep up our regimen until the first lockdown, when all the gyms suddenly shut. Desperate to maintain my fitness, I bought an exercise bike and some weights and continued to exercise at home, doing online classes.

But it wasn't the same. Without the discipline of going to the gym and attending a class at a specific time, it was easy enough to say, I'll do it tomorrow, or forget about exercise entirely.

Well, the gyms have now been open again since April and further restrictions were supposed to ease from Monday, so are things back to normal? No, not at all. Gyms are still operating at only half strength and remain hedged around with so many rules, regulations and restrictions that you wonder whether it is worth going at all. Opening hours have been drastically reduced and everything has to be booked in advance, even a session on the treadmill.

You are allowed to work out on the equipment for only 50 minutes at a time and you can book a maximum of seven sessions a week, whether these are classes or working on the machines. And you have to book. You can't just walk in and join a class or have a go on the rowing machine, as before.

All this has made many, if not most, former members feel that the gym is no longer good value and they have not renewed their membership. Nor are new members coming along.

The result is that whereas my gym was once a busy, bustling place, it is now sad and empty, and while there were once 20 or more people in the classes, the instructors are now motivating a multitude of three. Some classes such as pump – a weightlifting class - cannot be held because of the difficulty of disinfecting the equipment satisfactorily, or so it is alleged. Never mind that not a single case of Covid has been reported at my gym or, most likely, at any other.

I fear that the 'safety measures' which gyms have had no choice but to put in place have made many people scared to return even if and when all restrictions are lifted. I used to go to an 'old lady'. – ie, over-50s – Tabata class which was always packed. Not one of those old ladies, who used to live for their weekly workouts, has come back, even though this class has been once again on offer. Tabata, by the way, is a series of exercises each lasting 20 seconds, with 10 seconds off, and is supposed to be the most effective exercise regime ever invented. Pre-lockdown it was highly popular, but the management will not put on any new classes while numbers remain so low.

I am not blaming the gyms; they have to abide by government rules and guidelines, however ridiculous or unnecessary, for fear of being shut down if they do not conform. My gym, along with most others, has instigated a variety of online classes to compensate. But in much the same way that you have to go to church to get the full benefit of a religious service, you actually have to go to the gym, make the effort, join a class and have the motivation provided by an instructor at the front of the class, to retain maximum fitness. Sorry, but even the jolliest Joe Wicks class won't do it.

At the moment, neither our bodies nor our souls are being looked after, and without the gyms operating at pre-lockdown strength, we are gradually becoming a nation of porkers, fat and lazy, eating banana bread rather than putting in an hour on the cross-trainer. And regular workouts, as all exercisers know, are good for the brain as well as the body. I can sweat off much of my anger and frustration with a frenetic hour on the exercise bike. We've heard of 'runner's high', the adrenaline rush that comes from a satisfying run. I get 'biker's high' and the tingling sensation left by an intense workout lasts all day.

Regular hard exercise is good not only for physical health, it is also excellent for mental health, as all sportspeople know. I am not a swimmer, but I have several friends who have gone into deep depression because they have not been able to go to the pool. For many, especially the retired, their daily swim makes life worth living. And although most indoor swimming pools are now open again, a lot of people remain too frightened of catching Covid to return to lapping the lanes.

So, while purporting to 'protect' the nation's health by making us stay indoors, restricting exercise and sport, successive lockdowns have made us unhealthier than ever before and, paradoxically, much more likely to succumb to any infection going.

Without regular exercise, systems seize up and become sluggish, predisposing us to more illness and making us old and bent before our time. I also know that exercise works well for weight loss. One woman at our gym, before lockdown, lost three stone in a year on a regular exercise programme devised by her personal trainer. As a result, her confidence and self-esteem flourished. At the moment, there are no personal trainers working at our gym.

It is well known that as a nation we are suffering from an obesity epidemic. Boris Johnson has rejected a proposal to put extra taxes on sugar and salt, but a concerned move to get us all going to the gym, easing up all remaining restrictions and making sure they never recur, would do us far more good than all the test and trace, lateral flow tests, isolation, mask-wearing, distancing rubbish that is preventing a return to mental and physical wellbeing.

AUGUST 2ND, 2021

Keep those masks on!

IF I HAD HOPED THAT once mask-wearing became voluntary, people would be casting off their muzzles in their millions, I was very much mistaken.

Everywhere I go, people are still wearing them – in shops, on public transport, even on the streets and in their cars. Before we go any further, let me say that I abandoned my mask long before so-called Freedom Day on July 19th and I will never ever wear one again, unless of course I find myself in the unlikely situation of carrying out a surgical operation. And even surgeons don't always wear them these days.

Yet it seems I am very much in the minority, and sometimes even in a minority of one. One the very day that the mask mandate was lifted, out came the scaremongers, predicting that thousands of cases would result from this reckless act of tearing off the mask, that hospitals would be overwhelmed, and we would be back in lockdown before we knew it.

One of the most disappointing aspects for me is that many friends and colleagues I thought were intelligent, independent free-thinkers are campaigning for masks to be made compulsory again. An Oxford Community Association has started a petition to make mask-wearing mandatory and has asked people to sign.

Astonishingly, lots have done so. Many of my friends on Facebook have stated that they are pro-masks and will continue to wear them, even though they no longer have to. They maintain that by doing so they are protecting other people and other people are protecting them. It's complete rubbish of course.

Since the mask requirement ended, I have booked visits to art galleries and museums and well-meaning friends have said, 'It's crowded. Make sure you wear your mask.'

No fear! I don't even possess a mask any more. I have thrown them all away, both the used and the unused. Mind, I only ever bought the very cheapest and most useless, as my pathetic protest against wearing one at all.

But the self-righteous and the virtue signallers have come out in droves. For example, the Labour Mayor of Cambridge, Dr Nik Johnson, has issued the following statement: 'To keep our businesses open, and avoid more lockdown, I will wear a mask. To keep my colleagues and patients safe, I will wear a mask. I ask you all to join me.'

Now, Johnson is a medical doctor. Surely he understands that if you are not infected, you cannot infect anybody else. And the truth is that hardly anybody is infected.

When buying a pair of shoes last week, I saw this notice prominently displayed: 'In response to recent government advice, customers are no longer legally required to wear face coverings. Please note that for the protection of our community, store staff will continue to wear masks.' Restaurant and bar staff continue to wear them as well, creating a horrible distance between those who are serving and those who are served.

It gets worse. A few days ago I had a meeting at an Oxford college concerning a series of lectures that I am involved in this autumn. Everybody from the academic staff to the groundsmen and receptionists, was wearing a mask. Apart from me, of course. I was quite literally the only person in the college that day not wearing one. Try as I might, I could not persuade the others at the meeting to take their masks off while we were talking round a table. It was almost as though they were hot-riveted on. And they were fancy masks, too, not just the blue disposable variety.

Now that I am going around maskless, nobody says anything, although I do get some very odd and, I imagine, disapproving stares, although when somebody is wearing a mask, it is difficult to decipher their expression.

My hairdressers continue to wear masks and last time I was in the salon, I was the only client not wearing one. Once again, now that they are no longer compulsory, nobody could request me to wear a face covering, but they seemed uneasy about my bare face.

For me, there is every disadvantage in wearing a mask and no advantages whatever. For one thing I don't recognize people, even friends and neighbours. For another I can't properly hear what they are saying. We lip-read more than we realise, and as well as not being able to hear, I cannot read people's expressions. I can't tell whether they are smiling or serious, happy or unhappy, angry or pleased. Even worse, if I am wearing a mask in a shop, my glasses steam up when I am looking for something or trying to read a label. So, for me, wearing a mask in enclosed places means I can neither see nor hear. My lipstick smudges and on hot days, I start to sweat uncomfortably inside the mask.

Wearing one, not to put too fine a point on it, is a form of torture. Also, it completely wipes you out. Without a visible face, you lose all individuality and you might as well not exist. You have become a nameless, faceless peasant. And yet, in some circles these ridiculous and completely unnecessary face coverings have almost become designer accessories. You can get masks that match or co-ordinate with your outfit, and I have been dismayed to see Olympic competitors wearing masks when they are not competing. Nicola Sturgeon, Scotland's First Minister wears – wait for it – a tartan mask.

I despair. But even if I am making a unilateral stand, I will continue to go out and about mask-free in the hope that I am setting an example that others will follow. Otherwise, I fear, these face coverings will become so standard that nobody ever ventures out again without one. In the old days it used to be said that a lady was known by her gloves. Let us hope that in future she is not known by her mask.

What happened to responsible journalism?

WHEN THE AMERICAN ACTRESS Jennifer Aniston declared that she would 'unfriend' anybody who had refused the Covid vaccine or was an anti-vaxxer, she gained thousands, if not millions, of new fans who agreed with her.

Since then, others have stepped in to say that the unvaccinated are no longer their friends.

For me, it is just the opposite. I fear I am fast losing friends among the vaccinated, among those who proudly proclaim that they have not only been double-jabbed, but will be queueing to have the booster, so-called, that will be 'offered' in the autumn.

Have these people, I wonder, read anything about the vaccines, studied how they work and what they do inside the body? I doubt it. Even journalists, who are supposed to have inquiring minds, have no hesitation in condemning those who have chosen not to be jabbed even while admitting that they are ignorant about vaccines.

The latest was Hilary Rose, writing in The Times. Having stated that she knew nothing about vaccines, she went on to say: 'If the entire medical establishment says that something is for my own good and – crucially – those around me, then who am I to disagree?'

But Hilary, love, the entire medical establishment is *not* saying that these vaccines are for your own good. Far from it. All over the world, eminent doctors, scientists and virologists – those who actually do know something about vaccines – are questioning the efficacy and safety of these new, untried and experimental shots.

Hilary blithely ignores all this and instead denounces the 'rabid anti-vaxxer conspiracy theorists who foam at the mouth in Trafalgar Square.' Warming to her theme, she adds: They're beyond help and beyond contempt.' How can she be so sure they are 'beyond contempt' if she herself knows nothing about vaccines? Maybe it would be a good idea to mug up on the subject before castigating those who have the courage to protest against the imposition of an experimental drug on ever-younger members of society.

So the question I am asking is: why are we listening to such people as Jennifer Aniston, Sean Penn, Hilary Rose, *Daily Mail* columnist Amanda Platell and the ultimate loudmouth, Piers Morgan – none of whom know anything about the science of vaccination – and ignoring the research of informed doctors and scientists who are emphatically not 'rabid anti-vaxxers' and nor are they foaming at the mouth.

Instead, these scientists are presenting careful research in a calm and considered manner.

As a journalist myself, I used to be proud of my trade. I was given the opportunity to research and investigate many controversial areas, and report on them after I had amassed enough information to be able to write with some authority. I remember one fine journalist, Peter Martin, telling his employers the *Sunday Times* that he needed three months to research and write an article on cancer that was commissioned by his editor. As an old-school journalist, he wanted to get to the bottom of the subject before feeling confident enough to write about it.

All that has gone by the board since Covid reared its hydra head.

I have yet to read an informed, properly researched article in the mainstream media about coronaviruses, how they work and how they are best treated. But no, that is too much like hard work. How much easier and better to castigate all dissidents as nutjobs and crackpots without for a minute listening to what they have to say.

It seems that the louder you shout, the more you will be believed. The still small voice of truth is being drowned out while these ignoramuses – and I use the word in its literal sense – are allowed massive coverage in all sections of the media.

Let's vaccinate the world

WHEN I ASKED MY YOUNGER son whether he and his family had to take Covid tests before travelling to France, he replied, crossly: 'We are going for two weeks of swimming, lazing on the beach and relaxing, not worrying about whether we have to have tests.'

That's me put in my place, then. But while some people who would normally travel abroad, such as myself, have decided to stay at home this year, it seems that nothing will separate many members of the middle class from their foreign holidays. As I write, friends, colleagues and family are in Italy, Crete, Croatia, France and Greece, in spite of all the restrictions, tests and quarantining required for the pleasure of sunning themselves on a hot beach.

While the Taliban rampages through Afghanistan, foreign secretary Dominic Raab is on a 'luxury break', as the newspapers have it, in Crete. Piers Morgan, who has railed incessantly against the unvaccinated and unmasked, is even further away, in Antigua, for the second time this year.

For me at least, going abroad at the moment is simply not worth all the ridiculous and expensive tests required. Nor do I wish to keep the highly lucrative Covid industry going or to add to its considerable profits.

Vaccine-manufacturer Pfizer made $3.5 billion profit from Covid in the first three months of this year and the forecast is for $26 billion to be made by the end of 2021. Professor Dame Sarah Gilbert, one of the developers of the Oxford AstraZeneca vaccine, and widely hailed as a saint, is likely to receive a £22 million windfall when the company she created in 2016 floats on the US stock market later this year.

As vaccinations go further down the age range, the greater the profits will be.

At the moment, you have to be fully vaccinated to be allowed to go to France. My son and his family were not permitted to go until their 18-year-old daughter, my granddaughter, had been double-jabbed. Whatever you might think of the suitability of the vaccine for youngsters, there was no way round it. Unvaccinated children over 12 and under 18 would have to present a negative test result taken less than 48 hours before travel, never mind that they are probably completely healthy and have never had the virus or been anywhere near it. If you want to go to Italy, you need to have a negative test and must also call the Covid-19 helpline when you arrive. The NHS card, apparently, is taken as proof of vaccination.

None of this necessarily applies to the jet set who can fly around in private planes without any need for tests, vaccine certificates or self-isolation. They don't have to check in at airports or join a lengthy queue while their vaccination/PCR test status is checked. Nor do they have to wear masks while on board their planes, as lesser mortals do.

So, rich celebrities who continue to fly around the globe are putting two fingers up to the rest of the populace who have no choice but to abide by the restrictions or stay at home.

What it comes down to is that at the moment, those who travel abroad are not only keeping the whole Covid industry alive and making money hand over fist but making sure the restrictions are retained for the rest of us. For the more that people fly in and out of the country, the more we are warned that they could be bringing in or taking out a variant, whether or not this has any basis in truth.

Hence all these tests and protective measures, so-called.

Just out of curiosity, I did a quick online questionnaire for HALO, widely advertised as being the 'best test kit on the market.' I was advised that one double-vaccinated adult would need to purchase a HALO double pack for £159 to travel to France. And that was just answering the questions for one adult. Four such tests would add £636 to the cost of the holiday.

And at £159, the HALO test is not even the most expensive. A small company called Mayfair GP, which is government-approved, is charging £399 per test.

But are these tests even necessary in the first place? David Livermore, a medical microbiologist at the University of East Anglia, told *Mail Online* on August 10 that they are not. He said, 'There is little justification for the present level of pre-or post-travel testing.'

The tests may be completely unnecessary for travellers, but they are very good news for the providers as there is a huge mark-up on them. Professor Livermore reckons that the tests should cost no more than £20 and even at that price the manufacturers would make a profit. But it is all lovely jubbly, as Derek 'Del Boy' of *Only Fools and Horses* might say and getting lovelier all the time.

Don't expect our government, or any other government, to take notice of those who question the necessity for these tests, or to lift travel restrictions any time soon. So long as people insist on travelling abroad while countries are traffic-lighted as red, amber or green, these tests will not only remain but will very likely become even more onerous and expensive. Why kill a goose that keeps laying such golden eggs?

The only protest we can make just now is to holiday at home and not add to the huge profits presently being made by the Covid companies for the sake of a fortnight in the sun.

I am certainly not queueing up at an airport or forking out for any of the expensive and currently compulsory tests. I will stay put and save my money for – hopefully – better times ahead.

Service without a smile

IN HIS *TCW DEFENDING FREEDOM* article on Friday, September 3, Sean Walsh drew attention to the 'cancellation of the human smile' thanks to everybody wearing masks. Wherever I go, I still see the majority of people wearing masks, even though they are no longer compulsory. I am usually the only maskless person on the bus or in supermarkets. Just before entering a shop, most customers, young and old, get out their masks and put them on. I have even seen quite small children wearing them. And now, it is reported that 'ministers plan stronger guidance on wearing masks amid concern over falling compliance.'

As a result of still having to wear masks, staff in shops no longer offer service with a smile. Because of this, it has started to feel uncomfortably like you are being served by a robot. When nobody is able to smile, there is nothing to cheer you up when you are out and about.

But this whole mask-wearing nonsense, and the lack of smiling that goes with it, doesn't just wipe the humanity out of human interaction, it actually predisposes to mental and physical illness, as a number of scientific studies have shown.

Many years ago, I wrote a book called Smile Therapy, which took in all the latest research around then about the effects of smiling and laughter, not just on ourselves, but on those around us. I have just dug the book out and its message seems more relevant than ever.

In 1906, a French scientist, Israel Waynbaum, wrote a book called *Physionomie Humaine: Son Mechanisme and Son Role Social*, in which he postulated that facial muscles act as ligatures on the blood vessels and regulate blood flow to the brain. The blood flow in turn influences how we feel. From this, he developed the theory that emotions often follow from facial expressions, rather than the other way round.

When we smile, he believed, the increased flow of blood to the brain is associated with a healthy body and a positive mood. Sad and miserable expressions, by contrast, result in a decreased flow of blood to the b rain that can result in physical ill-health.

The different facial muscles that are used for smiling, anger, disgust and so on, all connect to different neurotransmitters in the brain which in turn send chemical messages throughout the body.

The act of smiling, theorised Waynbaum, affects all these brain hormones to their betterment and helps to keep people well and happy. His book was buried and forgotten about for many years, but a group of American scientists rediscovered it in the 1980s and decided to put his theories to scientific test.

They asked some actors to look in turn happy, sad, disgusted and surprised. As each expression flitted over their faces, instruments recorded changes in heart rate, skin temperature and blood pressure.

31

They found that far-reaching physiological changes accompanied each facial expression, even though the emotions they represented were only simulated. With the negative expressions, all body systems were hyped up and on red alert, but when the actors smiled, heart rate decreased, blood pressure went down and a state of relaxation ensued.

The results of these experiments showed that smiling and laughter have a vital part to play in the maintenance of health and the avoidance of illness.

The therapeutic value of smiling does not just lie with the person who smiles. There is an infectious element to smiling and laughter that can change the mood of those around us as well. People who smile a lot are not just keeping themselves well but helping others. Smiles oil the wheels of social life and offer friendship. When people like each other, they smile. The happier and wider the smile, the more pleased people re to see each other.

It has also been found that smiling is the only universally recognised facial expression and that it can be deduced from a far greater distance than other expressions. It might be difficult to tell, at least from afar, whether somebody is sad, disgusted or angry, but we can always tell when a person is smiling. When strangers smile at each other, this means: I come in peace. A smile will immediately put the other person at their ease yet if somebody approaches with a grim or threatening expression, the fear factor ramps up.

Smiling is, after all, the first 'human' expression that a baby produces, and parents are always keen not to miss that first smile.

It tells you that the baby is happy, not in pain and is recognising another face. The usual reaction when a baby smiles is to smile back, which is difficult if you are wearing a mask.

Apart from all this, smiling is a potent beauty treatment. When people smile, only one major facial muscle is used, whereas lots of muscles are needed to twist the face into negative expressions such as those of grief or anger. Smiling keeps people looking younger, while all other expressions are ageing.

If we keep wearing masks, or if a mask mandate is reintroduced (which would not surprise me at all) we may even forget how to smile and thus will remain strangers to each other, forever distanced.

It is not too much of an exaggeration to say that the fear of Covid, which keeps being stoked up, is exacerbated by mask-wearing obliterating the human, friendly expression of smiling. The less we smile, the more we are likely to become anxious and afraid, which in turn leads to succumbing to illness.

Never forget the old song:

> Pack up your troubles in your old kitbag
> And smile, smile, smile.

It could be the most potent message for our times: never underestimate the impact of a wide, friendly smile and in order to keep smiling, ditch that mask.

Smile Therapy: How Smiling and Laughter can change your life, published by Optima, 1987.

Yet more mask nonsense

HONESTLY, I DESPAIR. I really do. Five months after the mask mandates ended, not only are more people than ever wearing them in my part of the world, including small children, but we are increasingly being bullied into stringing them on.

The other night I went to a lecture at an Oxford college to find that at least 95 per cent of the audience of several hundred were wearing masks. At a book launch a few weeks ago (yes, I get around!) at least half of the attendees were wearing masks. Even if they took them off once they sat down, they walked in wearing them.

The request 'Please wear a face covering' had started to appear on bus tickets and some people I thought were intelligent are now saying they won't get on a bus any more because some of the passengers are not wearing masks.

The Transport for London website says: 'You must wear a face covering on the Transport for London network, in stations and for the whole of your journey.' Although masks are not compulsory on trains, National Rail have said that they still expect passengers to wear them throughout their journey. I'm sad to say that the majority comply. The level of compliance, in my view, is beyond belief and against all sense.

Queen Letizia of Spain has recently been photographed wearing a white mask at a gala event. The nauseating captions said: 'Queen Letizia shows off her impeccable style' and referred to her 'glorious' tiara. How can you look impeccable and glorious when you are wearing the kind of mask doctors use for surgical procedures? You just look ridiculous.

Boris Johnson was widely castigated for not wearing a mask when he was sitting next to 95-year-old David Attenborough. I don't have much admiration for the way Johnson has conducted the whole Covid farce but when I thought he was finally leading the way, he was condemned for not showing more respect for the ancient broadcaster, rather than admired for casting off the muzzle at last.

Most shop staff are continuing to wear masks and when I, mask-free of course, tell them that they don't have to, they reply that they 'choose' to. Some of the bolder ones tell me they have read the science. If that is really the case, they clearly haven't read the same science that I have, which says that masks are not only useless to prevent the spread of disease but that they actually make you ill. There is even a condition called maskne, a form of acne caused by constant mask-wearing.

As ever, 'the science' is conflicting. A report from the Cato Institute issued on November 8, 2021, entitled *Evidence for Community Cloth Face Masking to Limit the Spread of SARS-CoV-2: A Critical Review* has found there is no clinical evidence for the efficacy of face masks. The report concludes: 'Examination of the efficacy of masks has produced a large volume of mostly low to moderate quality of evidence that has largely failed to demonstrate their value in most settings.'

Yet if you read the good old Guardian, you will see apparently opposite findings. A report last Thursday by health editor Andrew Gregory cites a global sltudy published in the *British Medical Journal* which he says, has found that mask-wearing cuts Covid incidence by 53 per cent.

But what on earth is 53 per cent? How did Gregory arrive at such a definite figure which the *BMJ* in any case, does not use? In fact, the *Journal* hedges its bets by saying: 'This systematic review and meta-analysis *suggests* that several personal and protective measures, including handwashing, mask wearing and physical distancing are associated with reductions in the incidence of Covid-19.' (My italics)

The operative word here is 'suggests' and from that we can conclude that the findings of this so-called 'study' are vague in the extreme. But of course the Guardian pounced on it with the same relish that it has greeted all repressive measures, adding with glee that mask-wearing has been re-imposed by the Dutch government and that Romania, the Czech Republic, Slovakia and Poland have tightened their mask-wearing rules.

This *BMJ* report was also trumpeted by the Times, another publication which eagerly seizes on any excuse to reimpose or continue the use of muzzles and which underlined its stance by featuring a photo of Queen Maxima of the Netherlands wearing a mask.

The mask manufacturers, naturally, are laughing all the way to the bank. From March to December 2020, 224 billion masks were made in China. That was the equivalent of 40 masks for every person in the world outside China, and the figures must have vastly increased since then. In Brighton the other week I saw a whole shop window full of masks; glittery ones, designer ones, masks to match your outfit and masks in which to cut a dash.

When I go into a beauty salon, there is a box of masks at the entrance and I am offered one. When I say I am exempt they accept it of course but they are all wearing masks themselves. Doctors' surgeries and medical clinics also have boxes of masks for patients who walk in without one.

My audiologist admitted that all this mask-wearing is causing immense stress to the deaf and hard of hearing, who rely on lip-reading. Yet he is wearing one himself, never mind that every single one of his patients has a hearing problem, otherwise they wouldn't be there.

My younger son and I had lunch in a restaurant recently and I would say that we were the only customers who did not come in wearing a mask. My son became embarrassed when I fixed the wearers with my usual basilisk stare, shaking my head at their stupidity. When a masked person addresses me, I say loudly: 'I'm sorry but I can't hear what people are saying when they are wearing a mask.'

It makes no difference. They carry on wearing them.

What's wrong with people? Far from wanting to cast off their muzzles, breathe properly and become recognisable once again, they seem to be hugging their chains, or their masks, more than ever. A few years ago, there were campaigns in many countries to make hijabs and other face coverings worn by Muslim women illegal. Now, there are even renewed campaigns to make face masks compulsory again. We are all, willingly it seems, wearing hijabs.

That is, except for me and the other brave souls who refused to be tyrannised into wearing a face covering, as masks are euphemistically termed. I am just so disappointed that we appear to be in an ever-shrinking minority. If we are not careful, these masks will become the norm and our children will grow up in a world where nobody has a face, long after all real or supposed threat of Covid has vanished.

Mask mandate re-imposed!

FIRST OF ALL THERE WERE the supposed covidiots, those independently-thinking individuals who refused to believe that we were in the midst of the most dangerous pandemic in history and would have to cower in fear for the rest of our lives.

Now it seems that we have the 'maskidiots'; the brave souls who refuse to obey the mandate re-imposed on the nation on Tuesday, November 30th, 2021.

Leading the charge is Sir Desmond Swayne, the Tory MP for New Forest West, who in October said that the face-covering obsession could be dangerous to mental health because 'masks cover friendly expressions.'

Now he has gone further. He told Julia Hartley-Brewer on TalkRadio that he refused to wear a mask because of his 'genetic predisposition to liberty.' For this, he has won an award for 'the most idiotic excuse for not wearing a mask.'

Let me say here that I am with Sir Desmond, one of the few politicians who is talking any sense about mask-wearing. I too have refused to wear a mask since July, when the mandate was lifted and now that it has come back, I am still refusing to cover my face.

Why? I too believe that mental health can be seriously impaired by never seeing a human face and that if the entire nation continues to wear a mask we will see an epidemic, not of Covid, but of severe mental illness. Already, formerly cheerful friends are telling me that they are feeling depressed as never before.

Apart from that, I doubt that mask-wearing makes the slightest bit of difference to any infection going round. So many friends and colleagues who have obediently masked up everywhere they go have tested positive for Covid and some have come down with serious coughs and colds whereas I, who have never taken any notice of any of the restrictions, remain perfectly well. Mind, I am often told that I am made of stainless steel, which may be true.

I know in my bones that wearing a mask, especially when it's a dirty piece of cloth, offers no protection and may even predispose you to illness. Cloth masks in particular are pretty much worse than useless, according to a study originally published in the *British Medical Journal* in 2015 and updated to take in coronavirus advice. Such improvised masks, the study says, should not be regarded as PPE (Personal Protection Equipment) as they can actually cause illness.

And would you believe it, you can now get woollen balaclavas that have a zip for covering the face, thus turning them into a mask. They may be ideal for robbing banks (except that there are no banks open nowadays to rob) but they are pointless as defences against infection.

Prolonged mask-wearing, as demanded by some jobs, can cause actual physical illness as well. One *TCW Defending Freedom* reader, midwife Mary Stewart, wrote to the British Occupational Hygiene Society for clarification on the health risks of microfibre shedding from day-long mask wearing. Mary's son had developed a sinus infection severe enough for him to attend A&E caused, she believed, by his having to wear a mask for nine hours a day. The doctor said that he was seeing a lot of this, all Covid-related.

The fence-sitting response Mary received from the BOHS said that health risks from mask-wearing were concerning but they had not yet reached firm conclusions.

My home in Oxford is close to several schools and I am profoundly dismayed to see pupils of all ages wearing masks in the street. Gaggles of teenagers talk to each other through their masks. And I was also distressed to see a picture of Jacques and Gabriella, the six-year-old twins of Prince Albert of Monaco, wearing masks as they hugged each other.

The fear level has been ramped up so much that a friend who lives on the Isle of Wight said he was on a beach by himself when an elderly lady walked past wearing a mask. He said there was nobody else in sight!

I can state here that since last Tuesday I have been going out and about with a bare face (apart from make-up of course) to test the water, as it were. As a precaution I bought a pair of mask-exempt badges and downloaded an exemption card in case I was confronted, and this has happened only once.

As I walked into a shop, one customer asked rudely: 'Where's your mask?' I told her I was exempt and the woman behind the counter asked to see proof. I showed her my badge and said that I also had an exemption certificate in my wallet. She accepted these exemptions and agreed to serve me but I was told it was the law that anybody exempt must display proof by wearing their exemption on a lanyard round their neck.

But is it the law? The latest information from the Government website, updated on December 2nd, states plainly that you are exempt if you cannot wear a mask because of physical or mental illness, if wearing one causes severe distress or if you rely on lip-reading.

Further on it says that you do not need to show written evidence or an exemption card. I quote: 'Carrying an exemption card or badge is a personal choice and is not required by law.'

It is legally enough, then, to state that you cannot wear a mask, and so far, nobody has asked to see my exemption card or badge. The *Metro* newspaper, distributed free in the London area, splashed in its edition of Friday December 3 that 152 passengers travelling on public transport had been fined, another 125 were turned off the bus or tube, and another 5,100 told to cover up, according to Transport for London.

Speaking from my own experience, I took the coach from Oxford to London without wearing a mask. The driver said they had been told not to be confrontational and not to turn passengers off the bus for not wearing a mask. On a London bus I was the only maskless passenger and nobody said anything. If you look confident and are reasonably well-dressed, you are likely to remain unchallenged, as I am discovering.

As it happens, my own mental health has been adversely affected by the ridiculous mask-wearing imposition. For many years I have suffered from tinnitus and no longer hear very well.

I simply can't make out what people are saying from behind a mask. This has been causing immense stress as I have to strain to hear every word. In any case a mask will not fit if I am wearing my hi-tech hearing aids. What with glasses as well, there is simply too much going on behind the ears. One friend said she lost one of her hearing aids when trying to put on a mask on the underground and as the aids cost around £5000, it was an expensive loss. But for trying to put on the mask, the hearing aids would have stayed in place. I'm somewhat ashamed to say that the word schadenfreude came to mind.

As for me, even if I did not have a hearing problem, I would still refuse to wear a mask, out of principle.

So, far from regarding Sir Desmond Swayne as a 'maskidiot' I applaud him as possibly the only politician talking sense right now. I'm joining you, Sir Desmond, in the hope that ever more or us will walk the streets unmasked and restore some kind of sanity to the country.

The current mask mandate is supposed to be lifted on December 21. Will it happen? I have my doubts.

———

Update: Desmond Swayne retained his New Forest seat for the Conservatives at the 2024 General Election. Although critical of much Covid policy, he stated that he was an enthusiastic vaxxer, so my support for him is limited. See later for evidence of severe harm from the Covid vaccines.

———

JANUARY 17, 2022

Scotland the not so brave

AS NICOLA STURGEON ANNOUNCES THAT the Scots may have to wear facemasks 'for years to come', all I can say is how glad I am that I don't live in Scotland.

Since the new mask-wearing rules were introduced on November 23, I have refused to wear one and touch wood, fingers crossed, have got away with it.

In that time I have been on buses, coaches, the London Underground, stayed in a hotel for three days over Christmas, been to the cinema and to the hairdresser, the beauty salon, nail bar and in many shops and supermarkets, blessedly mask-free. I have taken taxis all over the place. Only once have I been apprehended, and that was in Sainsbury's, where a member of staff came up to me and asked, 'Where is your mask, madam?' I told him that I was medically exempt and he nodded and went away.

In the hotel where I was staying over Christmas, there were signs everywhere saying that masks were compulsory and that anybody not wearing one would be reported to the authorities. Yet I did not wear one, nobody said anything and nor was I reported to the authorities, whoever they might be.

It is true that on buses I have been on the receiving end of some nasty stares, or as nasty as they can be when most of the faces, and thus the expressions, of the other passengers, are hidden. It is also true that some people edge away from me as though I have got a deadly plague. My next-door neighbours, masked up to the eyeballs even when walking down the street, asked why I was not wearing a mask and I gave them the same response: 'I am medically exempt.' That, so far, has precluded further questioning although the truth is that I have exempted myself. I have no actual doctor's exemption although if challenged, I have an exemption card in my wallet, which I downloaded from a government site and which I can produce if demanded. So far, nobody has asked to see it.

The government website states quite plainly that if wearing a mask causes undue distress, you can exempt yourself from wearing one. In order to drive home the fact that I am not wearing a mask, I make sure I am wearing bright red lipstick every time I leave home. That way, I am making a clear statement that I am defying the rules and showing in no uncertain way that I am proud to be mask-free.

We were warned that we could face on-the-spot fines of £200 if we refused to wear a mask on the London Underground. Since the end of November, I have taken the Tube many times, always maskless, and have never been confronted or asked to see proof of exemption. I decided that if I was fined I would refuse to pay it and go to prison for my principles if it came to that. I would be a martyr for the cause! But none of the Underground staff has said a word and nor have any of the passengers. True, there are signs all over the place saying that masks are compulsory, both on trains and in stations, but I have just taken no notice.

The sad thing is that I seem to be in a minority of one. Everywhere I go, I am the only person, child or adult, who is not muzzled. It is monstrous that all secondary school pupils and children over the age of 11 have been told to wear masks in public indoor venues and on public transport. My neighbour, employed by Oxford University, says that she is required to wear a mask for work, even though on most days she is the only person in the office. She also has to keep taking tests.

Actually, I am going further than not wearing a mask. I have never had a PCR or lateral flow test, not had the booster and am not going to have it, either, in spite of Sir Chris Whitty telling me in the cinema that I must have it to protect myself and others. There are huge posters at bus stops and ads in every newspaper telling me to get jabbed, but I ignore them all. And guess what? I have remained completely well, not had so much as a sniffle throughout all this so-called pandemic, while just about everybody I know who has had the jabs, the boosters, the tests and who never dares venture out without a mask, has had Covid or what passes for it. Most of my refusenik friends, the few I have left who are defying all the strictures, say the same.

The mask mandates in England at least are due to be reviewed on January 26th but if they are relaxed, as I expect them to be, I will place a bet here and now that the majority of people will continue to wear them and tell you that it is their choice. Such is the state of fear that governments don't need to impose rules or threaten us with fines and imprisonment. We have become so cowed and terrified that we are imposing them on ourselves.

I just wonder how many people will be brave enough to defy the First Minister in Scotland, if she carries out her threat to make her compatriots wear masks for ever more.

———

Nicola Sturgeon was Leader of the Scottish National Party and First Minister of Scotland from 2014 to 2023. In the May 2024 General Election, the SNP were all but wiped out, losing 39 seats and holding on to just nine.

———

Those who see . . .

WE ALL KNOW THE STORY of the Emperor's clothes and the fact that a small child, rather than the courtiers and the sycophants, blurted out the truth, that the Emperor was, in fact, wearing nothing at all.

That story by Hans Christian Andersen was first published in 1837 and now, nearly 200 years later, its message is more relevant than ever. For while politicians, scientists and supposedly learned people everywhere were ordering us into lockdowns, pushing us to take ever more vaccines and tests, to sanitise our hands at every turn and to wear masks, it was the ordinary people who saw through all this and rebelled.

From the start my cleaners, who started a domestic services company after the hotel they had been managing was sold, realised that the wool was being pulled over their eyes, big time. Although several of their clients insisted that they wore masks and gloves when entering their homes, they knew in their bones that these measures were not only completely unnecessary but if anything, injurious to health. I told them that masks were forbidden in my home and that I would refuse entry to anybody wearing one.

Two make-up artists I know were also convinced that we were being spun a load of lies. One of them, Kim, not only puts as much dissident stuff on Facebook and other social media as she can get away with, she has also been on marches to protest against lockdowns and mask mandates. Indeed, she has conducted a ferocious campaign against mask-wearing which she knows, as well as do most scientists if they are honest, that these paper nappies, as she calls them offer no protection whatever against respiratory infections and are just a means of muzzling us up.

Kim is always being sent to Facebook jail for 'spreading misinformation' but as soon as the ban is lifted she is back there with ever more evidence of the great harm that Covid strategies the world over have caused.

My other make-up artist friend is convinced that vaccines caused, or at least contributed, to the death of her 19-year-old son. She risks being demonised as an anti-vaxxer but stands her ground. 'I know what I know', she maintains.

Such people, while perhaps not formally well-educated, have proved that they are independent thinkers, perfectly able to do the research and join the dots, while the supposedly clever ones, those with fancy degrees and posh jobs, persist in following the mainstream narrative to such an extent that they are now queuing up for their fifth jab and continuing to take those ridiculous PCR tests.

I live in Oxford, which for about a thousand years has been at the forefront of philosophical and scientific enquiry. You might expect an ancient university to be questioning government policy at every turn, but no, they have slavishly adhered to all the mandates and have even introduced extra restraints of their own. I am told that Cambridge has been even more hidebound in going along with Covid policies. It is doubtful whether these policies have saved a single life, rather the reverse, as there is mounting evidence that they have contributed to a larger than average number of deaths over the past two and a half years. But it seems that the cleverer you believe you are, the more likely you are to refuse to see or admit what is staring you in the face.

Most doctors have, of course, been compliant, with the result that the minority who have had the courage to speak out have risked being struck off. The handful of politicians who have questioned lockdowns and vaccine mandates have met with hoots of derision from their fellow MPs.

It is the same story in every profession and the higher up the ladder the individual is, the more likely he or she has attempted to dragoon the rest of us into going along with whatever nonsense Professor Neil Ferguson, Sir Chris Whitty, Sir Patrick Vallance or any other government advisers have decided to decree. Every time the country appears to be getting back to normal, another 'variant' is apparently discovered and the latest is that experts (whoever they may be) are warning of a 'triple-demic' this winter. The best advice is to take no notice of them.

Lord Sumption, who attained the uppermost reaches of the judiciary, has been pretty much a lone voice of reason among his peers in speaking out against Covid directives.

Meanwhile, senior journalists, broadcasters and editors are still bullying us to get vaccinated. Such people, generally speaking, have never studied the science of vaccines and have no idea what the spike protein, an ingredient of the Covid jabs, might be doing inside the body. Nor have they bothered to find out. Instead of discovering for themselves, they are demanding that we anti-vaxxers, as they call us, are forcibly silenced while they continue to assert, against all the fast-mounting evidence, that adverse side effects from these vaccines are rare, mild and fleeting.

As I started with the familiar tale of the Emperor's new clothes, let me finish with a Bible story, once again concerning a young child who saw the truth. Samuel was brought by his mother Hannah to assist Eli, the elderly priest of Israel, in the temple. Eli was asleep and Samuel eventually realised it was God speaking to him directly. The scene is captured in this children's hymn:

> *Hushed was the evening hymn*
> *The temple courts were dark*
>
> *The lamp was burning dim*
> *Before the sacred ark.*
> *When suddenly a voice divine*
> *Rang through the silence of the shine.*
>
> *The old man meek and mild*
> *The priest of Israel, slept.*
> *His watch the temple child*
> *The little Levite,kept.*
> *And what from Eli's sense was sealed*
> *The Lord to Hannah's son, revealed.*

The hymn finishes with these lines:

> *That I may read with childlike eyes*
> *Truths that are hidden from the wise.*

And didn't Jesus say that out of the mouths of babes and sucklings shall come wisdom?

The moral here is: instead of taking notice of those in positions of power who pronounce from on high, let us hearken to the ordinary people in all this, those who have no vested interests in keeping us fearful, cowed and miserable or in pushing harmful vaccines on us. They, like the child in the Emperor's clothes story, are the ones whose voices should be heard.

'Hushed was the evening hymn' was written by James Drummond Burns, a Scottish minister of religion and a poet. He died in 1855 aged 41.

Modern medicine has a lot to answer for

WHEN PEOPLE ASK WHETHER I have had 'my' booster and I tell them no and that I wouldn't dream of it, invariably the next question is: 'Are you an anti-vaxxer?' While asking this they often back away as if I have some deadly plague.

My answer – although these questioners don't want to listen to it – is that of course I am in favour of medicines that work and which don't do harm. But there is ever-mounting evidence that the mRNA vaccines do cause harm, as the tragic stories of severe vaccine damage attest.

And the jabs don't even protect you against Covid! Most people I know who have had the vaccine, and some have had up to five jabs now, have caught Covid, sometimes badly.

Just last week I was talking to somebody who said that she had refused all Covid vaccines but that her husband had gone along with every one of them. She told me that they both caught Covid, and with equal severity. Her husband's jabs did not protect him in the slightest. I doubt if this couple are an isolated example. Maybe I am just lucky but in spite of never taking a single precaution against Covid or flu, I have remained completely free from all respiratory infections for the past three years when Covid was supposedly raging, and much longer.

Ever since I began studying health and medical treatments in the 1970s I have learned that modern medicine is littered with apparent miracle treatments that either don't work or which do serious harm.

Does anybody remember the old Camel cigarette ad, which alleged that cigarette smoking was good for health, and stated that more doctors smoked Camels than any other brand? And Craven A cigarettes were promoted as being good for your throat: 'For your throat's sake, smoke Craven A.' The first scientists to produce evidence that smoking was actually bad for health and could cause cancer as well as other serious diseases, were laughed at. It was years before they were taken seriously.

Thalidomide was a dramatic example of a drug that did harm, as evidenced by the 'thalidomide babies' who were born with fingers attached to their shoulders and other serious deformities. Once again, the drug company manufacturing thalidomide, originally prescribed for morning sickness, defended their product in a huge fight, which made newspaper headlines. Finally the Distillers Company, which produced the drug, admitted defeat but it was a close call.

Since then there have been many other prescribed medicines that were enthusiastically welcomed and then later found to do more harm than good. I am thinking particularly here of benzodiazepine tranquillisers such as Librium and Valium. When I was a young mother in the late 1960s and early 1970s most of my contemporaries (although not me) were on them.

How they blessed these 'mother's little helpers' as the pills enabled them to get through the days of screaming babies, sometimes abusive husbands and mourning for their lost careers or the careers they were never able to establish. They sailed through their lives in an eerie calm and all seemed fine until they tried to off these prescription drugs. Then the fun started. Although marketed as non-addictive, these pills in fact were highly addictive and those who had been taking them found that withdrawal was by no means easy.

They reported that they had to wear sunglasses to watch television as suddenly, everything was too bright, but even worse, all the pains and mental anguish that had been kept hidden with the tranquillisers, rose to the surface. The problems had not gone away but had been buried deep by the pills. In some case the dependence had become so severe that patients had to be hospitalised or go into rehab.

The addictive potential of benzodiazepines was bad enough, but it paled into insignificance beside the effect of OxyContin, a morphine-based slow-release painkiller prescribed to millions of Americans. The full story of this dangerous drug, formulated by Purdue Pharma, a company owned by the Sackler family, is well documented in the award-winning, closely researched book *Empire of Pain* by Patrick Radden Keefe. The scandal was also aired on the Disney+ channel under the title *Dopesick*.

Doctors were bribed to prescribe Oxycontin by slick salespeople offering incentives such as a case of vintage champagne or exotic holidays. The Sacklers tried to redeem themselves by funding art galleries and university departments, much as rich families in Renaissance Italy became patrons of the arts after robbing everybody blind.

What made the OxyContin story particularly dreadful was that many of the Sacklers were doctors themselves. Profit was all and the Sackler family netted many billions from their aggressive promotion of what was basically heroin.

The point I am making here is that it is very difficult to trust medicines which yield profits beyond most people's imagining. In my lifetime I have never known a medical treatment to be so intensively pushed as the highly lucrative Covid vaccine, not just by doctors and scientists, but by most branches of the media as well. Anything that is so relentlessly plugged should be arousing suspicion, but so far we dissidents are not only in the minority, but are silenced and cancelled whenever possible.

If I wanted to book a face-to-face GP appointment just now, it would probably be impossible and yet I have received endless texts to go for my vaccine. In vain do I reply that I am not interested. They simply don't hear. Perhaps the reason for their sudden deafness is that they get paid extra for administering the jab: £12.58 per patient, and this is on top of their salary of £81,000 a year on average. If a GP surgery administers 60 jabs in a day – easily done as they only take a minute – that adds up to a handy extra £754.80. In a five-day week this bonus comes to £3,774.

The Conservative Woman website has published some excellent explanatory articles about what is in the Covid vaccines and how they can wreak havoc throughout the body. Many of these have been written by my ex-husband Neville Hodgkinson.

I take notice of what he says as he studied vaccines for decades in his capacity as a national newspaper medical and science correspondent, in the days when journalists took pride in telling the truth.

History, and especially medical history, has shown us time and again that when enormous sums of money and profit are involved, we must be very much on our guard and treat extravagant claims and endless reassurances with the scepticism they deserve.

The writer who deals in truth – and finds it hard to get published as a result

IF THERE WAS ANY JUSTICE in the world, American novelist Laura Sharrow, who writes under the name L.S. Sharrow, would be a best-selling author. Her fast-paced murder mysteries, featuring husband and wife private detectives Gina Slotkin and Paul Loya, and written mainly in dialogue, are real page-turners. Even though they are about murders, there are touches of throwaway humour throughout, and they are also short, unlike some of the impenetrable doorstopper thrillers which unaccountably rise through the best-seller lists.

With all this going for them, why does Sharrow have to publish her novels independently, under the radar so to speak?

It's because of the themes, which tackle anti-Semitism, trans men and women, homeopathic remedies and, slipping down very easily, a history of Israel. Sharrow is Jewish and so are many of her characters. But being Jewish is not the main reason she can't get published by traditional outlets: after all, many world-class authors are, and have been, Jewish.

No, she is cancelled or ignored thanks to going against the current woke grain with just about everything she writes.

For instance, two of her recent novels, Moxie and Hot Town, tackle the forced transition of children and teenagers. In Hot Town, a young Jewish transman is trying to detransition and become a girl again after being prescribed puberty blockers and undergoing a double mastectomy. Of course, the detransition will work only up to a point, as much irreversible damage has already been done. The male voice, for instance, brought about by cross-sex hormones, will remain all her life.

This character was put on to puberty blockers at 13, when she realised she was lesbian and attracted to other girls. Told by doctors and psychiatrists that she was trans, she understood too late that she was not, after all, 'trapped in the wrong body'.

Sharrow says, 'In these two novels, I deal with the medicalisation of children, with anti-Semitism as a backdrop. But I have discovered to my cost that it is impossible to get traditionally published with anything that criticises trans treatments.

'I also found that Amazon have been removing authors they regard as transphobic. I had a short story accepted by a mainstream publisher but when they learned of my opposition to medicalising gay and lesbian youngsters, they pulled the story. Since then I came to understand that most publishers will not go near an author who is opposed to children transitioning. Once I realised that, I decided to publish independently with my first and then second novel.'

She decided after those two novels to avoid writing any more about trans matters as they were just too unacceptable in the present climate. Her third novel, Savage, in which the detectives investigate the murder of an elderly Jewish woman, is more directly about anti-Semitism and is set in Paris just after the Charlie Hebdo shootings.

The story here is that on January 7, 2015, two Algerian Muslim brothers killed 12 people working on the satirical magazine, and injured 11 others, for printing a caricature of the prophet Muhammad. Two days later, a kosher supermarket was targeted on a Jewish holy day.

Sharrow does not pull any punches, and one of her characters in **Savage** says that Gaza schoolteachers tell their pupils that Israelis drink the blood of Muslim babies. A Muslim taxi driver is very rude to Gina Slotkin, the Jewish detective, telling her that he will not tolerate any insolence from women.

But this theme is not the only one to offend today's mainstream publishing business. In the same novel, homeopathic remedies are favourably featured. This undoubtedly upsets Big Pharma, who have for a long time denounced homeopathy as quackery and tried their level best to get it outlawed.

Sharrow, who suffers from ME, says, 'I have been immeasurably helped by homeopathic remedies when conventional medicine could do nothing. My son, now 49, had a persistent ear infection cured by homeopathy when orthodox medicine failed him. Yes, there are charlatans in homeopathy as there are in all branches of medicine, but I know from my own experience that it can, and often does, work.'

As one might guess, Sharrow is also vehemently opposed to the mRNA jab, and is firmly with Robert F Kennedy Jr on the forced vaccination of babies and children. On mRNA vaccinations and the matter of children transitioning, she says: 'They are both methods and technologies employed by Big Pharma and, in the case of transitioning kids, surgeries as well. If the idea, the plan, behind the jab was to depopulate, then an easy way into starting the process would have been through medicalising confused kids, kids with autism and gay and lesbian teenagers.'

She adds: 'At first I thought it was all about Big Pharma profits, but now I think it's much more sinister. Young people who transition are automatically rendered sterile. They also become lifelong medical patients. Massive numbers of young people have been made infertile through the mRNA jab. And they're beginning to drop like flies.'

Although Sharrow's novels deal with controversial themes and murders most foul, they are a light, sometimes comic, read and among the light relief is the investigative journalist Nigel Harrison, an amusing and affectionate depiction of the late writer Christopher Hitchens. He himself was Jewish, something he learned only at the age of 38 after his mother committed suicide.

Throughout history, it has been the subversive voices in the wilderness that have eventually led to the truth coming out, and Sharrow's gift for plot and witty dialogue constitute the latest brave salvos against the forces of darkness which threaten to engulf us.

L.S. Sharrow's Gina Slotkin murder mysteries Moxie *and* Hot Town *are available on Amazon on Kindle and as e-books, and* Savage *will be available after March 27, 2024.*

Let us remember the Stoics

THE STOICS OF ANCIENT TIMES believed that in many cases it was possible to control pain by thought alone. To achieve this, they stoically, as it were, accepted painful or unpleasant sensations, viewing them with studied indifference. As such, the pain often went away of its own accord, although to be fair, they did use a painkiller known as theriac, which contained opium.

The opposite is also true, in that you can induce pain or disease by thought, causing acute and sometimes lasting physical symptoms. Although ancient and tribal societies understood that the power of suggestion can be so strong that it may make people ill or well, this seems to have been forgotten in modern, mechanistic medicine with its insistence on tests, scans, screens and so on.

Because of this, I am now wondering whether so many people would have gone down with Covid (or what passed for it) if, instead of a flu-like illness being ramped up as the worst and most dangerous disease ever to affect humankind, it had been ignored.

As it was, around 80 per cent – and it may have been more – of the world's population were gripped by such a fear of the bug that they actually thought themselves into illness. Once the PCR test was introduced, people began testing themselves, sometimes hourly, and if the test showed positive, they waited for symptoms to appear. More often than not, the symptoms obliged.

Then people began to be terrified of stepping outside the house without wearing a mask, even though all the evidence showed that these muzzles were more or less ineffective and that even the surgical quality ones only offered protection for a couple of hours; the length of time they are usually worn in hospital theatres. People also began to be nervous of getting close to anybody else, edging away if somebody came within a few feet of them. Only the other day, as I was in a queue waiting to pay for an item, a masked woman in front of me turned round and said crossly, 'Do you mind not standing so close to me?' I wondered about making a quick riposte but decided that there was no way I could penetrate this kind of stupidity.

There was also the handwashing ritual where shops, doctors' surgeries, solicitors' and estate agents' offices, for instance, forced hand sanitiser onto you and sometimes took your temperature as you walked in.

The cleaning nonsense went even further, with hotels, gyms and other places where people gathered announcing 'enhanced cleaning.' This may or may not have halted the virus in its tracks but it certainly increased fear. I still see people in the gym furiously scrubbing down bikes, treadmills and other equipment in case a germ from a previous user has had the audacity to linger on the machine.

I also remember, during the first lockdown, a friend invited me for a drink and insisted we sat in the corridor to her flat, holding our glasses while wearing surgical gloves. She would not let me into her home and she also paid her cleaner to stay away. I of course had no such fears but I could persuade very few people to step over my threshold while lockdowns were in place. Delivery men rang the bell and then ran away sharpish so as to remain 'Covid safe.' There has never, in my lifetime, been anything to compare with the fear and terror that has gripped the world – and all for a largely harmless threat.

When the vaccines were introduced, people eagerly queued for the jabs, but did this make the fear go away? No, it increased it to such an extent that they lined up for ever more jabs. I know people who have had five injections and ended up in hospital with severe pneumonia. But still they have praised the vaccines, telling themselves and others that, but for the many injections, their symptoms would have been so much worse. Never mind that, by and large, the unvaccinated, for which read fearless, remained perfectly well throughout. In my view, the fear created the milieu which allowed the infection to take hold in the vaccinated.

Now of course, we know from many studies that the vaccines themselves are harmful but try telling that to the multiple-jabbed. Their fear has taken such a grip that they refuse to listen, and these same people are now booking their spring and summer 'booster', so that they will have had perhaps six or seven jabs by the end of the year.

The friend who made me sit in the corridor to have a drink had had all the Covid jabs plus the flu jab and guess what, she has been laid up for several days with quite a nasty infection. After she had all the jabs, she said: 'Now I'm protected.' Yes, so protected that she languishes in bed, unable to get up.

Why are people not putting two and two together? I think it's because they cannot bring themselves to believe in the power of the mind to create illness or wellness. The poet William Blake wrote in 1794 of the 'mind-forged manacles' by which he meant that we make these manacles for ourselves and we create a prison in our own minds which then becomes a reality. Once the mind-forged manacles get a grip, illness can result.

Over the past three years, we have created manacles, prisons, misery and pain for ourselves, aided and abetted of course by the mainstream media. And the fearmongering is far from over. Hanging over us all the time are threats of more lockdowns, more restrictions, more mask mandates, more jabs, more curbs on our freedom, all designed to keep us cowed and afraid.

Since 2020, when the first lockdowns were introduced, it has become clear that those of us who were unafraid, who resisted all the testing, masking, distancing, jabbing and other interventions, are the ones who have remained well. Our strong minds acted to strengthen the immune system and allow us to resist infection, as in the Latin phrase, *Mens sana in corpore sano*. A healthy mind in a healthy body.

The two go together and modern medicine ignores the power of the mind at its peril. We need to learn from the Stoics!

We are the martyrs of today

WHENEVER I GET OFF THE bus at Oxford city centre, I see the monument to the Oxford martyrs, Hugh Latimer and Nicholas Ridley, who were burned at the stake in Broad Street in 1555, and Thomas Cranmer, who suffered a similar fate the following year. The three refused to renounce their Protestant beliefs during the reign of Catholic Mary Tudor and died the most horrific deaths as a result.

I have often thought, when passing the monument and the commemorative plaque set in the wall of Balliol College opposite, that these men could have saved themselves simply by recanting, an option that was open to them and indeed, Archbishop Cranmer did recant before reaffirming his belief in Protestantism.

Now, I see more clearly that, whatever the consequences, they could not in all conscience revert to a faith they no longer held. We like to think we live in more civilised times and we no longer burn people at the stake for not conforming to the religious orthodoxy of the time – but do we? The history of the past three years has been an updated version of martyrs being consigned to the flames for their beliefs, but this time the rejected articles of faith are the Covid vaccines.

They have become the new religion, with fervent advocates even among church and spiritual leaders. Instead of enjoining us to believe in God, they have urged us to save ourselves by having the vaccine. Their sermonising on the matter has even acquired the status of holy writ as, according to Justin Welby, the current Archbishop of Canterbury, Jesus would have wanted us to have the vaccine. The Dalai Lama also urged his many followers to be 'brave and come forward to be vaccinated' after having the jab himself.

So, as the faithful line up for their sixth jab, the vaccine can be considered the secular equivalent of Holy Communion. The point of Holy Communion is to partake of the body and blood of Christ to absolve us from our sins, and the mRNA vaccine is supposed to protect us against bodily ills. In both cases, the idea is to keep the devil out by a ritually repeated observance.

Those of us who have done our research and cannot in all honesty believe in the magical power of the vaccine to ward off the devil of Covid infections, are the heretics of today who deserve to be burned at the stake, or in today's equivalent to be cast out of polite society and ridiculed as anti-vaxxers, conspiracy theorists, tinfoil hat wearers and covidiots. Doctors have lost their jobs for refusing to accept the supremacy of the vaccine and the very few politicians who have spoken out against it have been ostracised and marginalised.

Of course, when it comes to Protestantism or Catholicism, it is a question of belief. Yet we know how the vaccines work and have proof that they are harmful and can set up a variety of adverse reactions in the body. As such, those of us who know the truth cannot recant whatever the cost, as to do so would be to accept the lie that the mRNA vaccines have been a wonderful success story the world over, saving millions of lives.

But even as evidence of severe damage and sometimes death from the vaccine mounts up, as reported on *The Conservative Woman*, this continues to be brushed aside and even denied. Indeed, those who question the holiness of the mRNA vaccine to protect us from all ills do so at their personal and professional peril. Whenever a vaccine-related serious side effect or death is reported, it is dismissed in the media as 'extremely rare' and insignificant compared to all the good the rollout has accomplished.

And when a fully vaccinated individual catches Covid anyway, the believers' standard response is to allege that, for the multiple jabs, their illness would have been so much worse. Vaccines have become, one might say, the holy water of our times.

We may live in a largely secular age, but we have substituted belief in God for a belief in science, and most especially medical science, or what passes for it these days. We have come to worship Big Pharma with the same kind of adoring reverence we used to reserve for God and Jesus, and this persists even when the so-called science fails us.

The religious fervour goes even further. The ever-increasing number of vaccines administered to babies can be considered analogous to a holy baptism. For just as baptisms and christenings were supposed to cast out original sin before the baby had time to commit a sin, so today the many vaccines are supposed to cast out death in the shape of measles, mumps, rubella and chicken pox, or prevent them from entering in the first place. Once again, the supposedly protective substances are injected long before the baby has had any time to develop any of the infections.

Belief in the efficacy and safety of vaccines is so devout that nobody is allowed to raise a dissenting voice and anybody who dares to do so, such as Dr Andrew Wakefield, risks not only being discredited, but actually struck off the medical register and not allowed to practise. More recently, Dr Sam White was suspended for 'spreading misinformation' about the efficacy of the Covid vaccine. Robert F Kennedy, Jr, a challenger for the American presidency, is routinely attacked for promoting anti-vaccine propaganda. Yet to their eternal credit these people will not be silenced.

The search is now on to find a vaccine to combat every ill that flesh is heir to, including cancer and malaria. Living in Oxford, I am always getting alerts from the Oxford Vaccine Group to be a volunteer for one of their new studies. If vaccines cannot actually deliver eternal life, they can, we are led to believe, confer the next best thing, which is eternal health.

At one time, those who did not believe in God were considered wicked. Nowadays you are labelled an apostate if you don't believe in the almighty power of the vaccine.

So I wonder whether I would be prepared to concede, under extreme torture, that the mRNA vaccine was safe and effective. Thankfully, my conviction that it is neither has not been put to such a severe test but pondering on the issue has given me a new understanding as to why Latimer, Ridley and Cranmer were prepared to die horribly for what they believed was true, rather than recant to save their skin.

We know now that it was the sacrifice of these men, and particularly that of Cranmer, which made England a Protestant country. By the same token, I can only hope that those who have had the courage to speak out against the mRNA vaccine and who, because of this have been marginalised, ridiculed and in some cases lost their livelihood, will enable the tide to be turned at last.

Whatever happened to responsible journalism?

IT IS NOW 50 YEARS since I joined the Sunday People, a tabloid newspaper then selling more than five million copies a week, and that meant 12 million readers; about a quarter of the country's population at the time.

Our newspaper was a successful mixture of fun stories such as 'He's the biggest cat in the world and he's afraid of mice!' and serious investigations like the famous one about the laboratory beagles forced to inhale cigarette smoke. Although I was primarily a fashion writer on the paper I was also called on to take part in investigations and exposures. These were nerve-racking, often frightening assignments and we sometimes put ourselves in real danger, such as when one reporter entertained a murderer in her flat after his girlfriend had knocked her unconscious in a pub.

This same reporter (not me!) also had to pretend to be a prostitute for a story. She was sitting in a chair when the brothel owner came up, looked over her shoulder , saw that she was writing in a notebook and said: 'You're the first prostitute I've met with perfect Pitman's shorthand.' The reporter thought quickly and said that she used to be a secretary but couldn't make enough money at it. Sometimes you had to be quick off the mark to get yourself out of trouble.

My friend and colleague, the late photographer Doreen Spooner, was working at the Daily Mirror when the newspaper got a call that Christine Keeler and Mandy Rice-Davies were sitting opposite each other in a pub, and if the photographers were quick, they could get a picture of these 'two tarts'. The press photographers arrived en masse, but the pub landlord wasn't having any of this and refused to let any of the photographers in – except for Doreen, as there were very few female newspaper photographers in the early 1960s and it didn't occur to the landlord that Doreen might be one of this dastardly crowd.

Once in, she went straight to the ladies', worked out the exposure and quickly took a picture of the 'two tarts'. She was out of the door before the landlord realised what was happening. Not only did that picture make the front page next day but became world-famous and is still used in stories about the Profumo Affair.

Doreen said later that she was extremely nervous and knew that it was on the cards that the landlord would twig that she was a photographer rather than a customer and smash her camera.

Over the years, I reported, for various newspapers and magazines, on such subjects as dangers from tranquillisers, fluoride in water, alternative treatments for cancer, the success or otherwise of IVF treatments, the ethics of surrogacy and the efficacy of certain natural treatments. Editors allowed me to bring to the fore issues which were then in the shadows, such as domestic violence and child abuse. I was given freedom to write on controversial matters such as factory farming and NPK fertilisers and thus bring them to public attention. I also wrote about macrobiotic diets, vegetarianism and vitamins and minerals, at a time when any nutritional departure from meat and two veg was considered cranky.

Journalism was fun and exciting and we felt we were doing an important and responsible job. A particular skill that I had, I like to think, was to be able to read scientific, medical and academic papers and make them intelligible and accessible, even entertaining, to the general reader, without being patronising or dumbing down. I also explored esoteric subjects such as yoga and meditation, reincarnation and the paranormal.

Now, though, I am ashamed of the profession which I used to love so much and which gave me so much satisfaction. Instead of tackling tough subjects with honesty and open-mindedness, today's newspapers and magazines are full of endless fashion and cookery pages, plus celebrity gossip and royal tittle-tattle. Nothing serious ever seem to get a look in.

Over the past three years, not one mainstream outlet, whether print or broadcast, has mounted an in-depth, critical investigation of the Covid crisis and the hasty rollout of experimental and untested vaccines. Instead of politicians like Andrew Bridgen being given a serious hearing for raising concerns about vaccine damage, they are demonised as 'anti-vaxxer conspiracy theorists.' Not one major branch of the media has said of Bridgen: Hey, this guy might be onto something; let's listen to what he has to say. Similarly, not one mainstream outlet has taken a hard, serious look at Robert Kennedy Jr's book *The Real Anthony Fauci*, where he exposes the scientists and others peddling the highly lucrative

Covid and vaccine narrative as crooks and liars. Instead, Kennedy has been accused of 'misinformation'; never mind that his arguments are thoroughly backed up and he has not been sued.

It is true that some anti-lockdown commentators such as former Supreme Court judge Jonathan Sumption have been given newspaper space and airtime but no editorials got behind him, and no national newspaper ever instigated an anti-lockdown campaign. Yes, now that we have been freed from house arrest, they are asking whether the lockdowns were necessary or achieved anything, but none of them said a word at the time. Instead, we were bullied and cajoled into going along with it all, and woe betide any prominent person who dared to go out and about without a mask. No notice was taken, either, of all the reports and surveys showing that masks were either ineffective or downright injurious to health.

Even worse, celebrities were wheeled in to enjoin us to 'follow the science'. TV doctor Hilary Jones was saying as late as November last year that 'vaccines are the best way to protect yourself, friends' – a remark that was reverentially reported in the mainstream press. There was not one dissenting voice and this was at a time when people were known to be suffering, some quite badly, from vaccine-related illnesses.

Rather than being frank, fearless and free, as they boasted at one time, today's newspapers have shown themselves to be mealy-mouthed, timid and spineless throughout the whole episode. Most of the mainstream media are still alleging that vaccine damage is 'tiny' compared to the 'millions of lives saved', in the face of ever-mounting evidence to the contrary.

It has been left to brave and outspoken sites such as *The Conservative Woman* and *Daily Sceptic* to publish authoritative articles and to report the evidence which mainstream outlets have been afraid to publish. We can only be glad that so far is had been virtually impossible to impose total censorship on what one is allowed to say.

Yet headway is gradually being made, forcing important material to get into the public domain and doing the job that the mainstream should be doing.

It is also interesting to note that, whereas we journalists once prided ourselves on being ahead of the public, the public are now ahead of the journalists. The comments below the line on *MailOnline*, for instance, show that the public has a far greater awareness and understanding of what is going on as regards vaccine damage and the lockdown disaster than the journalists who are supposed to be the advance guard.

One can only hope that thanks to a few courageous souls relentlessly chipping away at the lies, deception and sheer falsehoods, the truth will eventually emerge and the media, which has so shamefully misreported this whole charade, will have the humility to admit how wrong they were and how they misled their readers.

If, that is, by that time they have any readers left. The *Sunday People*, once a mighty force in the land, now has a pathetic circulation of under 60,000. Perhaps that says it all.

How one brave man took on the mighty – and won

IF YOU HAVE EVER WONDERED why petrol used to contain lead before it was gradually phased out, you can thank one man, Professor Derek Bryce-Smith. His story shows how cool, evidence-based campaigning can eventually win the day, even when the whole world – or at least big corporations – marshal in all their might against you.

There are very close parallels here with those now drawing attention to the harm, serious illness and even death which has been caused by the mRNA vaccines and who are similarly being dismissed as cranks, conspiracy theorists and barmy anti-vaxxers. I am writing about the lead in petrol story to give hope to those who, like Mike Yeadon, Andrew Bridgen, Robert F. Kennedy, Jr and others voicing the truth and are not giving up, even in the face of countless attempts at character assassination.

My own part in Derek Bryce-Smith's story came about because, in 1986, I was working on a book about the many health benefits of nutritional zinc. Through a number of meetings as his laboratory at Reading University, where he was Professor of Organic Chemistry, I learned how lead additives in petrol came to be banned.

In the 1950s, Bryce-Smith, then a young researcher working at King's College, London, wanted to get hold of some tetraethyl-lead, which was routinely used as an 'anti-knocking' agent in petrol, for an experiment he was conducting. Tetraethyl-lead improved the efficiency of vehicles, turning clunky engines into smooth-running ones.

Derek looked through all the chemical catalogues at his disposal, only to discover that tetraethyl-lead was absent from each one. Wondering why, he wrote to the manufacturers, Associated Octel, and asked them to explain the reason. A representative from the company visited him to say that they did not normally make the stuff available, even to experimental chemists.

Why, Derek asked. The answer was that the stuff had dangerously poisonous qualities. 'It attacks the brain,' he was told. 'If you had an accident with it you could be killed or left insane.' The company's representative added: 'If this got out, the papers might try to get hold of the story and start saying we shouldn't add it to petrol.' The fact that King's College was very near to Fleet Street, then the heart of the national newspaper industry, might well have had some bearing on Octel's concerns.

Derek eventually persuaded the company to let him have some of the product after he explained the nature of the experiment he was working on – nothing to do with lead in petrol – but was warned: 'If you spill any on the floor, you will have to take the whole floor up, and if you get any on your finger, it will be absorbed through the skin and drive you mad or even kill you.'

Until then, nobody, including Derek Bryce-Smith, had questioned the need for lead to be added to petrol. An American chemist,

Thomas Midgley, had invented leaded petrol in the 1920s and insisted it was safe. All oil companies unquestioningly accepted this, and the production of lead additives for petrol became a highly lucrative worldwide industry.

But Derek got thinking – and researching. He discovered that the heavy metal lead could cause serious behavioural problems, particularly in boys, and could build up in the brain and the blood. A visit to a Henley-on-Thames hospital for autistic children confirmed this, as the blood in these children was found to contain extremely high levels of lead. Derek became the first person to draw attention to the health dangers of lead in petrol, and he was dismissed as a crank and a scaremonger for his pains.

One reason for his marginalisation as a crackpot was because so many chemists, particularly academic researchers, depended on the oil industry to provide them with money for their research and experiments. Sounds familiar?

Derek persisted, at grave risk to his academic reputation, and eventually the first clinical studies were conducted in 1960. They showed beyond all doubt that lead had toxic impacts on humans, and could stay in the system for ever, causing kidney damage as well as other serious illnesses. Once in the brain, lead could also impair intelligence and cognitive abilities.

Finally, notice was taken of the dangers of lead in petrol and it began to be phased out in the 1970s. Perhaps older readers can remember some pumps having leaded petrol and others containing lead-free fuel. Gradually, ever more countries began to ban leaded petrol and the last country to do so was Algeria, in 2021. Today, you cannot buy leaded petrol anywhere – and this is largely due to the pioneering work of Derek Bryce-Smith.

Now, adding lead to petrol is recognised as possibly the greatest experiment in mass poisoning ever undertaken. But even when the evidence became overwhelming, Associated Octel fought and fought for lead in petrol to be retained. They tried their hardest to prevent lead curbs eating into their profits, and they bribed at every turn, offering envelopes stuffed with £1,000 in cash, expensive holidays and other lucrative inducements to government officials. The company particularly bribed Iraqis to retain lead in petrol and were successful for many years.

Eventually, Octel had no choice but to cave in. Yet to this day, the company, which has diversified, maintains that lead particles in food and water are far more dangerous to humans than airborne particles from petrol vehicles.

Our book, *The Zinc Solution*, explains how zinc can work to drive out heavy metals from the system and improve all body functions. It recommends a simple, effective and cheap solution to many disorders which cannot effectively be treated by Big Pharma. The acceptance of zinc supplements as an important aid to health is once again largely due to Derek Bryce-Smith's work.

His story shows how one determined man can take on the industrial giants – and win. He had nothing to gain, financially or otherwise, from campaigning against lead in petrol. Rather, he had everything to lose, as his professorial job was on the line. But he persisted as he was determined for the truth to come out.

So I say to those now accumulating evidence of serious harm from mRNA vaccines, don't give up. Eventually the truth will dawn. It has to.

———

The Zinc Solution, by Professor Derek Bryce-Smith and Liz Hodgkinson was published by Century Arrow in 1986. Derek Bryce-Smith died of Parkinson's Disease on 11 June 2011, aged 85.

———

A medium-profile paedophile in our midst

IN COMMON WITH MANY JOURNALISTS, I was shocked and horrified to learn that Peter Wilby, former editor of the Independent and the New Statesman, and respected columnist and commentator on politics, cricket and current affairs, had been found to be a long-term paedophile, downloading over many years appalling images of children being sexually abused.

Although I did not know Wilby well, I took notice of his articles on university and secondary education as he was considered something of an expert, having been an education correspondent on a number of newspapers. He contributed a weekly article to the *New Statesman* until November last year and also wrote frequently for the *Guardian.*

Yet after I read the report of his conviction in the *Times* on Saturday August 19, a memory started to surface. This was that Wilby had written many articles saying that allegations of paedophilia were often witch hunts perpetrated against innocent people.

What I, and others, now realise is that all this time Wilby was hiding in plain sight and covering up his own paedophilia by exonerating others who had been accused of this crime. Why, he even castigated journalists who were investigating the claims made of sexual abuse in children's homes, saying they were naïve and, in hot pursuit of a story, often conveniently ignored the truth. Wilby drew comparisons to allegations of Satanic abuse which he denigrated as 'baseless conspiracy theories' and conjured up Dennis Wheatley-type images of evil monsters in black robes, presiding over child torture. No sensible person, the articles implied, could possibly believe such things went on.

Wilby praised a book by Richard Webster, an academic who had made an exhaustive study of abuse claims and concluded that many were without foundation and were maintained by public hysteria. Webster argued that there never was a paedophile ring at the Bryn Estyn boys' home in Wales, which was investigated by the *Independent*, and that the supposed perpetrators had all been falsely accused. Wilby supported Webster's theories all the way.

Dean Nelson, a journalist working on abuse allegations at Bryn Estyn for the Independent during Wilby's editorship, wrote on X (formerly Twitter) on August 20: 'As the editor of the *New Statesman*, Peter Wilby was the paedophile's friend. He ran articles denigrating victims as liars on the make. He sided with those convicted of abuse against their victims.

Nelson continued: 'Peter Wilby was one of my editors on the Independent on Sunday where I investigated the North Wales child abuse scandal. I was sued for libel by Supt. Gordon Anglesea, a senior policeman implicated as an abuser. He won, and three of my witnesses killed themselves. In 1998, Wilby became editor of the *New Statesman* and ran a piece criticising my investigation by Richard Webster, who campaigned for convicted paedophiles who, he claimed, were innocent victims. He claimed my witnesses were liars manipulated by me. Wilby never contacted me to offer a right to reply. When I complained that Webster was an apologist for paedophiles, Wilby said: 'You mustn't say that, it's not fair, he's a respected academic.' Journalist Bea Campbell also thought that Webster was an apologist for paedophiles.

'Gordon Anglesea was later convicted of the abuse my witnesses had accused him of, and he died in jail a few weeks later. All too late for my witnesses.

'Wilby had championed an apologist for paedophiles and now I learn that Wilby himself is a paedophile. He admitted a long-standing sexual interest in children and some of the images on his computer show real children being sexually abused. He was given a ten-month suspended sentence. No jail time for Wilby: he was a gentleman journalist after all. He should die in jail, for the abuse and the abuse of trust.

'It's no wonder paedophiles like Supt Gordon Anglesea felt above the law. They had champions like Wilby in their corner, shaping the debate.'

While the Lucy Letby story has received saturation coverage in every branch of the media, and the neonatal nurse who has been accused of killing seven premature babies was labelled as being so wicked that her lifetime prison sentence should mean life, there was hardly a word about Wilby following the short news report about his sentencing at Chelmsford Crown Court on Friday, August 18. For downloading horrific images of children aged nine to 13 being abused, which he admitted, Wilby was given the most lenient sentence possible: a ten-month sentence suspended for two years. He was also required to undertake 40 hours rehabilitation, be subject to a ten-year sexual harm prevention order and placed on the sex offenders' register for five years.

Adam Sprague, operations manager at the National Crime Agency, said: 'The material accessed by Wilby and recovered from his computer showed real children being cruelly and sexually abused.

'He was viewing this content while working as the editor of prominent news outlets, a role in which he was entrusted to form the news agenda for the British public. A trust which he has greatly betrayed.'

Pictures of Wilby coming out of court showed a pathetic, bent old man walking with a stick and wearing a raincoat. I don't know whether it was a dirty raincoat, but the convicted Wilby looked a far cry from the jaunty, confident journalist of yesteryear.

All this was faithfully reported, but there was little else from the media outlets which had published Wilby's articles. Toby Young came forward to write a Spectator column on Wilby's hypocrisy, later republished on his dissident website, *The Daily Sceptic*, on how he himself had been vilified by the man when he set up free schools. Wilby even accused Young of being a pornographer, the very thing he was himself. Police found 167 indecent images of children on Wilby's computer, stating that many were of 'the worst kind.'

Until he was arrested in October 2022, Wilby had covered his tracks so successfully that nobody suspected him of having a perverted sexual interest in children. His demeanour was that of an elder statesman, dispensing wisdom and well-reasoned opinion from on high. It seemed that he was a commentator to be trusted and nobody, at the time, wondered why he was writing so many articles about paedophilia, or what particularly interested him in this seedy subject.

So why, we have to ask, has there been so little coverage in the mainstream media about Wilby following his convictions? Why so little outrage? True, the Daily Mail's excellent investigator Guy Adams looked into Wilby's championing of paedophiles in a long article published on Saturday August 26, but no other branch of the media followed it up and there is continuing silence from the *New Statesman*, *Guardian* and *Independent*, the very media outlets which published so many of Wilby's pro-paedophile articles which, as Guy Adams pointed out, are still up on their websites.

Press Gazette, the journalists' online newspaper, owned by the same company as the *New Statesman*, repeated the news story, but did not add any comment.

And so far, Stephen Glover, one of the founders of the *Independent*, and a *Daily Mail* columnist, has not said a word about his former colleague. The story has, apparently, died.

Some people reckoned that the lack of coverage was because very few people outside the media would have heard of Wilby and while this may be a factor, had anybody heard of Lucy Letby before that scandal broke? Peter Wilby was far more high profile than she was when she worked anonymously as an NHS nurse. As well as being a prominent commentator on current affairs,

Wilby is also the author of a number of books, the latest being a well-received biography of Anthony Eden, the former prime minister.

I believe that the main reason the Wilby story has not attracted more comment is because the MSM are still protecting their own. After all, are the *Guardian*, *New Statesman* and *Independent* likely to admit they were very, very wrong to publish Wilby's articles exonerating paedophiles and accusing their victims instead? So far, the only statement from the New Statesman has been this: 'The *New Statesman* staff and management had no knowledge of Wilby's arrest or charges before they were reported yesterday and are shocked and horrified to learn of these appalling crimes.'

Dean Nelson, the journalist who first investigated allegations of abuse at Welsh children's homes, believes that the staff and management *did* know about Wilby, as he wrote so many articles accusing journalists of mounting witch hunts against purported paedophiles, but that they chose to say nothing.

It's good of course, that Wilby has finally been found guilty of downloading obscene images of children and that Guy Adams did a proper, traditional investigation into the former newspaper's holier-than-thou articles, as the *Daily Mail* headline had it. But while Wilby's articles remain on websites for all to read, paedophiles are still being protected.

I particularly remember one article where he wrote that non-relatives should be allowed to show children physical affection without being demonised by it, and thought it sounded creepy at the time. Yet I never twigged that Wilby himself might harbour a sexual interest in children; a perversion he admitted in court.

At the very least, the media outlets which published so many of Wilby's pro-paedophile articles should issue grovelling apologies for having misled their readers for so long. But will they?

Update: although Peter Wilby may have only been of medium profile, an extremely high-profile public figure was convicted of making indecent images of children, on July 31st, 2024. This was the television presenter Huw Edwards, he of the sonorous voice and serious expression when reporting, Dimbleby-like, on state and other important occasions. Edwards was handed a six-month sentence, suspended for two years, on 16 September 2024, at Westminster Magistrates' Court. This was an even lighter sentence than that handed down to Peter Wilby.

His crimes received blanket coverage because not only was he employed by the BBC which takes the licence fee by force but received a yearly salary of nearly half a million pounds. Edwards was also considered 'the voice of the nation' for his coverage of many royal occasions, such as the Queen's funeral, King Charles's Coronation and the funeral of the Duke of Edinburgh. As such, his broadcasts went all over the world.

Although this Peter Wilby story is not about Covid, it is yet another example of how today's supine media can cover up or simply ignore important stories if they care to. The Huw Edwards story received huge coverage because it enabled print media and other broadcast channels to take massive digs against the BBC, both for paying its 'talent' such enormous salaries and for not only continuing to pay Edwards after the scandal broke but even to give him a substantial pay rise. Now that he has resigned from the BBC, he will collect a pension of around £300,000 a year.

———

So am I a conspiracy theorist?

THIS TERM IS HURLED AT people as one of abuse but if I am so labelled, it is now because I am being awkward and contrary for the sake of it. It is because, having studied all the available data and research, certain conclusions as to what has been going on over the past few years are staring me in the face. I have, one might say, become awakened to the truth.

There is, so far as I am aware, no conspiracy involved in what I have come to believe. I am not 'conspiring' with anybody to spread misinformation for the sake of it, but simply making up my own mind having sifted through all the medical and scientific evidence, all the statistics and read very many books. And if my conclusions don't fit the propaganda being peddled by mainstream media, I will just have to remain out on a limb. For instance, although evidence is coming in from very many studies and statistics that the mRNA 'vaccine' does more harm than good, it is still toted as 'safe and effective' and is being rolled out as an autumn booster against a supposed new variant. And, I'm afraid, many people are queueing up for the new jab to 'protect' them against Pirola, or BA2.86, whatever that is supposed to mean, billed as the latest Omicron strain.

Fear has gripped them once again.

The real problem is that many, if not most, of those who adhere to the official narrative have done absolutely no research of their own. They just take as gospel what the mainstream media say, never delving any deeper or availing themselves of any of the wisdom of those who have diligently done their research.

One example stands out, but he is far from alone.

A few weeks ago a friend and former colleague came for lunch. As I hadn't seen him for a few years, naturally our conversation eventually turned to Covid and its ramifications. This friend, an Oxford graduate, qualified lawyer and film producer, had never heard of the World Economic Forum, Klaus Schwab, the Young Global Leaders, the Great Reset, *The Conservative Woman* website, the *Daily Sceptic*, Neil Oliver, Whitney Webb, Robert Kennedy Jr or anything or anybody pertaining to what is probably the greatest crisis to hit humanity, ever. Nor had he read any books, listened to any podcasts or watched any YouTube videos which asked awkward questions about the vaccine, lockdown, Covid tests, masking or anything else.

He had never heard of Anthony Fauci, Dr Mike Yeadon, Professor Angus Dalgleish. Dr Joseph Mercola or even former High Court Judge Jonathan Sumption, who from the start has questioned the legality of otherwise of lockdowns. In short, my friend had never heard of any of the expert dissenting voices which have been all over the networks since 2020. And yet, despite this ignorance, he had of course had all the jabs – six so far – worn a mask, taken the tests, obeyed lockdown rules to the letter, all without having the slightest notion of why he was blindly obeying the mandates.

He believed that the mRNA vaccines were 'safe and effective' without ever trying to out how they behave in the body, how they are made or what a spike protein is. And he is supposed to be intelligent!

I would like to say that he is the most ignorant person I have come across in these matters but that would not be true. He is just the most recent. Not long ago I was having a drink in an Oxford pub with a senior editor from a publishing company. This person has edited the works of many famous writers, but when I started talking about the Covid nonsense – try to stop me – she said she knew very little about it and quickly changed the subject. There was no interest whatever in trying to find out the truth, and this was from somebody who might be considered to have an enquiring mind. Once again, she is an Oxbridge graduate.

I'm afraid that ever since Covid-19 was announced in early 2020, the world has divided into two groups, them and us. Until we start talking, we don't know into which camp an acquaintance or relative might fall and the relief if we discover they are one of 'us' is overwhelming. For instance, I was a memorial event earlier this year and the photographer, a man I knew very slightly, came up to me and said, 'I've read everything on *Conservative Woman*, including your articles, and want to say I agree with every word.' This chap said that his mother was also one of us, and that they had done their research. I almost fell in love with him on the spot!

But sadly, it is always the same story. The 'thems' have never done any research or reading of their own, while the 'uses' keep up to date with every twist and turn of this devastating saga, bravely exposed by a few brave souls.

OCTOBER 1ST, 2023

An uplifting discovery

Sometimes, just sometimes, life takes an unexpected heartening turn. Just recently I was invited for lunch by a couple of friends I had known since university days but had not seen for at least a decade. I found Mark and Anna, both in their late seventies, looking extremely well and not remotely near their actual age.

After some initial chat and catching up, I wondered whether the dread subject of Covid, vaccines and so on, would be brought up and if so, who would broach it. On so many occasions when meeting old friends, I have hardly dared to mention it, wishing to avoid the barrage of abuse that might follow if they were unbelievers, members of the tribe of the unawakened. And as I have reported before on *Conservative Woman*, you never know in advance who might be one of 'us' and who might be one of 'them'.

In the end it was Mark who sprang the surprise, a pleasant one this time. He said: 'I read *The Conservative Woman* every day and I have seen your articles and Neville's, as well as those by other contributors.' He went on to say that he agreed with every word, and that he also reads five or six other dissident views before breakfast to keep himself up to date. He is a particular fan of Dr John Campbell. He also admires James Delingpole for his brave and uncompromising stand on the climate nonsense, vaccine nonsense and the way we have been comprehensively misinformed by mainstream media for many years. Mark and Anna are also major supporters of MP Andrew Bridgen, who has himself had to endure much abuse for his pronouncements that go against government policy.

Over lunch, this couple, who have been happily married for more than 50 years, explained that at first they had gone along with the official narrative. They obeyed lockdown, mask mandates and trotted along for their first vaccines. 'We were so careful,' said Anna. 'We sat outside in the cold with our children and grandchildren when we were told not to go indoors with them, and we regularly tested ourselves. We were, after all, elderly, possibly vulnerable and certainly did not want to be accused of being super-spreaders.

'We were taken in, one hundred per cent.'

Then, gradually, Anna said, the doubts started creeping in until they became converts, perhaps even going further than such as me.

Anna continued: 'Mark had been perfectly well all his life, but just two weeks after one of the mRNA vaccines, he suffered a stroke. It came completely out of the blue, with no warning. Of course, we cannot conclusively prove that the vaccine caused it, but we started to wonder, and then, for the first time, began doing our research. It soon became clear to us that the much-vaunted and highly pushed vaccines were neither safe nor effective, and that was when we decided we were not going to have any more of them.'

Now, both are completely disenchanted with the mainstream media and say they never want to watch or listen to BBC news any more. 'I used to be an enthusiastic listener of Today,' Mark said, 'but now I wouldn't dream of turning it on, for all the lies they have been pushing for the past three years or so, not only about Covid, but climate change, the Ukraine war and everything else that passes for news these days.' Mark reserved particular opprobrium for Greta Thunberg: 'How has this kid, who is not a scientist and has only just stopped being a schoolgirl, managed to inveigle King Charles, who called her 'remarkable' and also world leaders at the UN conference? None of it makes any sense.'

Anna and Mark are both very clever people who have had big careers and could now be enjoying an extremely comfortable retirement, but they say they have had all their previous ideas and certainties comprehensively shaken up. They are fervent Brexiteers and go along with *Conservative Woman* contributor Karen Harradine, who wrote in April that 'national treasure' David Attenborough has been one of the greatest indoctrinators of climate angst and has spent years traumatising children that the world is going to end. And yet Attenborough, as Mark pointed out, has flown all around the world and continues to do so with his expensive camera crew while enjoining us all to stop driving cars or heating our homes to 'save the planet.'

Mark's scorn for Sir Jonathan Van-Tam knows no bounds. Van-Tam is the UK's former deputy chief medical officer who has recently taken up a post as a senior medical consultant to Moderna, one of the companies churning out Covid vaccines. Mark asked: 'Did you know that Pfizer made 27 billion dollars profit from the vaccine last year? And the lies being spread by vaccinate-the-world Bill Gates, Anthony Fauci and Professor Chris Whitty, the chief medical officer for England, continue to astound me.' He added that he had signed the Great Barrington Declaration, drawn up by numerous scientists questioning the official response to the Covid outbreak and once again, rubbished by many on the orthodox side.

Anna says that she is most worried about what sort of world her young grandchildren might have, as I believe are all of us who have been enlightened and had our consciousnesses raised by the stalwart scientists, doctors, researchers and others who have relentlessly questioned the official narrative and opened our eyes so wide that they will never shut again.

It was heartening that Mark and Anna, dear old pals I have known for more than 60 years, think alike, because I have met many married couples who can no longer speak civilly to each other; one has seen the light and the other remains in the dark ages. It was also more than gratifying to add them to my list of true friends. As another friend remarked, 'There are more of us than people realise. It's just that until recently, so many have been afraid to speak out.'

My awakened friends, most of whom have now retired, say that the events of the past three years have given them a new lease of life, an important cause to fight for, when they might otherwise have eked out their days playing bridge, going round the golf course, doing crosswords or, worst of all, watching BBC News.

Now, some less heartening news

AFTER WRITING ABOUT THE HEARTENING experience with my old university friends who had seen the light after one of them suffered a stroke following a Covid vaccine, I have to report that this sadly is not the case with all my former friends.

Some weeks ago I had a communication from an old chum who used to live next door to us in Newcastle. We had not been in touch for perhaps 30 years but she had read an article of mine in a magazine – unrelated to Covid or such issues – and wondered whether we might be able to meet. She added that she had married again after her husband's death some years previously.

I said yes, I would be delighted to meet and catch up and we arranged to meet in Reading, a halfway point for both of us. But the day before she emailed to say that she and her partner had just had their Covid and flu jabs – their seventh Covid shot – and as a result she had become quite ill and could we arrange another date. That was OK by me, and I gave a few dates when I would be available. A few days later I had another email to say that her husband was now in hospital with a chest infection and she would be in touch again when he had recovered.

On another occasion, I arranged to meet somebody who had valuable information concerning a new book I was researching. We agreed on a date and venue, but the day before I got an email to say that his wife was in hospital and could we arrange another date. This we did, only for me to get another email to say that this time he had been taken to hospital with a very serious infection and would not be able to confirm when or whether we might be able to meet. Once again, they were fully up to date with their jabs, I was told, so were surprised to be laid low with these infections.

Sadly, these stories have become all too common since Covid, the vaccines and the PCR tests entered our lives. It has always been the case, in my experience, that the ones who succumb to an infection often serious enough to be admitted to hospital, are always, ALWAYS, those who have had all the jabs. I have never had a meeting cancelled by anybody unvaccinated throughout this whole episode.

Do these people not read *The Conservative Woman* or any of the other sites which have repeatedly told the truth about the Covid 'vaccine' and particularly the booster shots, which neither prevent transmission nor infection and are far more likely to do harm than good?

It is a fact that just about all the people I know who have had booster shots have been ill within days, in some cases seriously enough to require hospital admission. One friend nearly died after her sixth jab and it was touch and go in hospital for several days. Yet she still queued up for the seventh shot, plus the flu jab – and was ill again.

The other day I noticed a long queue of people outside my local branch of Boots. I asked one of them why they were all standing in line. He replied that owing to staff shortages, the branch was closed between one and two and they were just waiting for the shop to re-open. So what were they all queueing for? Yes, you've guessed it- the latest booster shot.

But why, now that Covid has gone away and whatever variants may still be hanging around are weak indeed? Maybe it's the pressure and the fear which is still being applied. Even though I have repeatedly told the NHS and also my GP practice that I am not interested in the shots, I still get texts inviting me to come for them. The latest, on September 18, said: 'You're a priority for seasonal flu and Covid vaccinations because of your age.' The text even said that they would come to my home if necessary. There was a link for me to opt out of invitations for 'my' vaccinations, but I decided to ignore it as, if I replied, they would then know I had read the message.

Given that my university friend cancelled two dates because of infections caused by the jabs, I am now wondering what more we can do. The evidence for serious harm from the vaccines is out there and has been for some time but all too few people, it seems, are heeding it. Would they rather become ill and have to be admitted to hospital than refuse these shots?

My neighbours have also obediently had their booster and flu shots and all have succumbed to infections since. In vain do I point out that I have never in my life had a flu shot, would not dream of having a Covid booster and have not had flu for at least 50 years. More to the point, I have never had Covid or even the slightest sniffle since the lockdowns, mask mandates and social distancing – none of which I have obeyed – began in 2020. Nor have I ever taken any of the Covid tests.

If I had expected that my own continuing excellent health throughout the Covid years, without taking a single one of the precautions advised or imposed, might make the jabbed among us take notice, I could not have been more wrong. They prefer to regard me as some sort of irresponsible loony who has just been lucky.

What WILL it take to overturn the nonsense?

PS – I never did meet up with my friend and her husband. A later email told me that her husband was now in a wheelchair and that travel was difficult if not impossible for him. We eventually spoke on the phone. And all thanks to these booster shots that are supposed to confer health, not illness.

Sometime later I had lunch with an old friend, and she is an old friend, 93, and now living in a care home. Naturally our chat eventually turned to Covid and I asked whether she had had the jabs. 'Yes, of course,' she said. 'I've had them all, plus the flu jab. Are you telling me that you haven't had any of the vaccines?' When I told her that I wouldn't dream of having them she looked at me in utter disbelief. 'You must have a very strong immune system then,' she retorted. 'I've had all the jabs and all the boosters with no adverse side effects at all.' And yet, she told me that she had been having panic attacks and had completely lost her appetite.

Her doctor, she said, had put her on anti-anxiety pills and they made things worse, if anything. Now obviously I can't say, and nor can anybody else, that the attacks were a side effect from all the vaccines, but I wouldn't be surprised as she told me she had never before suffered from these attacks, nor had she ever lost her appetite. True, she is in her 90s, but as a former world traveller and travel writer, she now says she cannot walk the few yards to the café where she used to have lunch every day.

We are the ones who remain polite and good-tempered

It's a strange fact that while believers in the official Covid narrative, now being given another indulgent airing by the Hallett Inquiry, have abused and vilified the dissidents, we have been unfailingly polite and courteous to our detractors.

To take the latest example, Carl Henegan, Director of the Centre of Evidence-Based Medicine at Oxford, was called out for talking 'half-baked nonsense' for his questioning of the lockdowns and other disastrous Covid policies. By dramatic contrast, he remained restrained and professional in his own responses. In her account on *The Conservative Woman* of the Covid Inquiry, Dr Ros Jones remarked on the way that Sage, Whitty and other mask and vax proponents, have been praised for their efforts, while the word 'f*ckwit' was used to describe Professor Henegan. Even Baroness Hallett,who is conducting the Inquiry and is therefore supposed to be impartial, barely managed to be civil to him.

Andrew Bridgen MP has been castigated for drawing public attention to the excess deaths since Covid entered our lives and as we have seen, most of his fellow politicians voted with their feet by their non-attendance when he finally secured his debate on the subject. Never mind that Bridgen's speech was full of closely-researched data and evidence, barely any of our elected Members of Parliament deigned to listen to it.

This was an occasion where pictures spoke more loudly than words, as the cameras panned round the almost empty House. Yet Bridgen did not comment, at least publicly, on the sheer rudeness and bad manners of this fellow politicians who failed to attend or walked out. He just gave his speech calmly but forcefully to those few seated around the benches.

Those of us who, while less in the public eye, have questioned the official narrative from the start, have also received our fair share of abuse. We have been called conspiracy theorists, tinfoil hat wearers and dangerous peddlers of misinformation. We have had our Facebook posts taken down, our X (Twitter) accounts suspended and often become alienated from family and former friends for questioning the 'science'. A friend, 'one of us' says that the mildest rebuke she has received is 'you're so boring these days.' Others in her circle tell her that she has gone crazy from living on her own, and that is why she has embraced so many lunatic theories.

We have been stigmatised as armchair or amateur doctors, scientists and epidemiologists, as if we are not allowed to investigate and research for ourselves. Of course, the worst insult we have had to endure is to be called an 'anti-vaxxer.' Piers Morgan railed on television against the anti-vaxxers, calling them 'not just half-wits but quarterwits.' He and others have spared no calumny is denouncing us, never asking whether we might have a point, or good reason, for refusing to be jabbed.

When I tell my detractors that without taking any of the so-called Covid precautions I have remained perfectly well, with not even the slightest sniffle, they come back with: 'The reason you have stayed well is because all the rest of us obeyed restrictions, self-isolated, took tests, worn masks and had every booster. We have protected you.' It has proved a complete waste of time to point out that it is mainly the vaccinated ones who have gone down with respiratory illnesses of one kind and another following their seventh or eighth booster while most of we unboosted ones remain unscathed. If we demur, we are told that it was since lockdowns, masks and bans on social gatherings were lifted that Covid has let rip once again. 'I know people who have died from Covid or are suffering from long Covid' we are informed, if we dare to point out just how badly the economy, businesses, education, mental and physical health have suffered, and for no good reason, since restrictions were imposed.

Even though evidence of harm from the mRNA vaccines is accumulating all the time and becoming hard to ignore, we are still being called super spreaders, crackpots and granny killers for not going along for the latest booster. One highly boostered person I know recently went down with Covid and 'it's grim, very grim' she pointed out, blaming it on the fact that nobody was wearing a mask on the Underground.

Those brave souls who have set up and run dissident, ie, truth-telling, websites have had their Twitter accounts suspended, their bank accounts stopped and their advertising withdrawn, in a concerted attempt to demonise them and shut them down. They have faced unspeakable character assassination. But still they have carried on, refusing to be silenced.

Yes, our opponents have been nasty to us. They have reached for the vilest insults they could muster. They have done their worst. Over the past three and a half years I, along with many others, have endured more insults for the stand I have taken over the Covid nonsense than at any other time in my life. But we have not returned insult with insult. We have just got on quietly with writing articles, holding talks and events, going on peaceful demonstrations, doing whatever we could to uphold the truth and make our voices heard.

We get their backs up because they are frightened of us, but the paradox is that our detractors' sheer loathsomeness towards us is having the exact opposite effect that they intended. Why, on Facebook just the other day a one-time believer in the official narrative posted oncologist Professor Angus Dalgleish's paper on the increased number of cancer relapses he has been seeing since the mRNA vaccines were introduced, commenting: 'This is interesting.' Well – possibly even thanks to the relentless raining down of insults – people are finally starting to wake up and take notice.

Update: Andrew Bridgen was the Conservative member of parliament for North West Leicestershire from 2010 until 2023, when he was expelled from the party for criticising the efficacy of the Covid-19 vaccine. He joined the Reclaim party but resigned in December to become an Independent. Sadly, he came second from last in the May 2024 General Election, securing only 1568 votes, and therefore lost his seat. He continues to campaign against the vaccine. Bridgen has a degree in Biological Sciences.

DECEMBER 8, 2023

How Covid changed me

WHEN I SAY THAT I have never been the same since the Covid debacle I am sure I am speaking for very many people. Before the first lockdown of March 23, 2020, I was bumbling along, writing articles and books, going on foreign holidays, meeting friends for lunch and dinner, going to the gym several times a week and pretty much enjoying life.

Since then, life has changed so dramatically, and generally for the worse, that I am sure it will never return to what it was. All of a sudden, measures were introduced that had never been seen in peacetime and were rigidly enforced. Our previous freedoms, taken for granted, were severely curtailed. We had to wear masks, distance ourselves from family and friends, even when we were perfectly well, and told to test ourselves regularly for the presence of a hitherto unknown and deadly virus. The most alarming aspect of all this was not so much that so many citizens accepted these restrictions, but we actually baying for more.

In December 2020, the first vaccine was rolled out in the UK and we were coerced into taking it. In some instances, it was compulsory to have the jab if you wanted to continue in your job, to travel or to be admitted to hospital. Television presenters such as Piers Morgan and Andrew Neil, while knowing nothing whatever about the make-up of the vaccine or what its effects might be, condemned those who declined it as halfwits or quarterwits. They went further, thundering that refuseniks should be denied medical treatment for putting everybody else at risk. When were we last forced to have an untested, experimental medication which had no discernible benefit and could cause great harm?

Now, four years on from Covid being touted as a new and highly infectious respiratory virus in November 2019 and the worldwide fear and panic which was induced as a result, my previously comfortable little existence has been aroused out of its torpor. The main reason for this is that some very uncomfortable truths have forced themselves on me.

Among them are:

1. In so far as I thought about them at all, I assumed that the World Health Organisation and the United Nations were benign institutions promoting peace, goodwill and health for all. Now I know that they are the complete opposite and are among the most corrupt outfits in the world;

2. I regarded Bill Gates as must a technology whizzkid, even though his Microsoft technologies, on which he had got the world to depend, were always going wrong and never worked anything like as well as the hype. Now I know that, far from being a benign philanthropist, Gates is a sinister Bond-type villain for real, who wants to depopulate and rule the world. His Bill and Melinda Gates Foundation has given vast sums to print media and television channels to ensure their compliance. Meanwhile, he has got his sticky fingers firmly and very lucratively into the pharmaceutical

industry. Thanks to donations of huge sums running into millions, the mainstream media have not dared to utter a negative word against him. Instead, they have run many sycophantic articles and interviews. It has been left to the brave dissident sites, always in danger of being defunded and shut down, to tell the truth about what is really going on with the Gates Foundation and its various offshoots;

3. The pharmaceutical industry, far from being dedicated to making us healthy and well, is mainly invested in illness, as that is where the profits lie. They want to get us all on drugs, preferably for life, as there is no money in a well person. This means that we must be constantly tested for this and that illness, given multiple injections and if possible put on medications such as statins for life. None of these medications make people well. At best, they may prolong the agony, as many have severe long-term side effects. Meanwhile, natural remedies, such as Vitamins C and D, fresh air and exercise, have been denigrated as 'unproven.' My realisation is that most pharmaceutical preparations not only do not cure but often make things worse. Yet they are heavily advertised everywhere, the latest being for a vaccination against shingles shown at every cinema in the UK. There is some evidence to suggest that the Covid vaccines encourage shingles to develop and certainly I have known several people who have developed this painful condition after one or other of the Covid jabs. Whether or not there is a link, I just don't trust the industry any more, and I now steer very clear of all medications, doctors and hospitals;

4. Politicians are largely in the hands of lobbyists and donors, who naturally attach conditions to their donations. If

I had previously suspected this, I now know it to be an incontrovertible fact;

5. Covid restrictions and mandates have served to divide society and friends and families, in some cases beyond repair. Maybe that was the plan all along – to restrict gatherings and make us wear masks and isolate, so that we were marooned in our own tiny spaces, unable to connect with others and exchange ideas as we once did. The shutting down of schools, universities and business places enabled this isolation, and working from home of course intensified being shut off from our fellow humans;

6. Climate change, or at least man-made climate change, is pretty much a scam and as much a money-making exercise for a few elites as Covid and the pharmaceutical industry. Yes, the climate is always changing but I now believe that the human input is minimal. Once again, thanks to so many scales falling from my eyes, I have been able to research the climate controversy for myself, and without having to take undue notice of the likes of David Attenborough and the ever-grinning Chris Packham, BBC luvvies who, indirectly at least, benefit from Gates money;

7. Once, I was happy to use cards instead of cash, believing that this system of payment was easier and more efficient than carrying around wads of notes. When Covid stalked the land, cash was considered dirty, as it had often passed through many hands, some of which might have been infected with the virus. As such, it was being cynically phased out on spurious health grounds. Cards were cleaner and gradually, ever more restaurants and businesses became 'cashless' or 'card only'. It then dawned on me or, more accurately,

was pointed out, that debit and credit cards enable every transaction to be monitored, whereas cash is less easy to track, and that this was the real reason for trying to do away with the folding stuff. So now I get wads of cash out from the bank and never use cards if I can help it. Once again my eyes have been opened as to what is really going on and that is: control;

8. Finally, I have come to the conclusion that we have been taken for a massive ride by politicians, lawyers, scientists, doctors, civil servants and international institutions and it has taken Covid to make me realise it. So perhaps some good has come out of it, after all.

JANUARY 15, 2024

We would true valour see

WHEN I WAS A CHILD, we often sang John Bunyan's hymn, *Who Would True Valour See*. I have to say that although I quite liked the tune – *Monk's Gate* by Ralph Vaughan Williams – the words meant very little to me. What was 'true valour' and who on earth wanted to be a pilgrim anyway?

Along with many youngsters of the day I was given *Pilgrim's Progress* as a Christmas or birthday present and was terrified by George Cruikshank's illustrations of the monster Apollyon, Faithful burning at the stake and Christian with the burden on his back sinking into the Slough of Despond, climbing the Hill Difficulty and descending into the Valley of Humiliation.

But since the Covid, climate change and now Post Office debacles, the force of Bunyan's hymn, first published in 1687, has finally come home to me.

Let's have a look at the words. I am using Bunyan's original version written in 1684 rather than that amended in the early 20th century by Percy Dearmer, who reckoned that hobgoblins and foul fiends were not suitable for Christian hymns.

Here is the first verse:

Who would true valour see
Let him come hither
One here would constant be
Come wind, come weather.
There's no discouragement
Shall make him once relent
His first avowed intent
To be a pilgrim.

Those of us who have true valour and as a result come hither are the growing numbers who have seen through the lies, misinformation and sheer wickedness peddled by the mainstream media, drug companies and the many doctors and scientists who have adhered to the official narrative and pulled a great deal of wool over our eyes. We have braved far more than mere discouragement for telling the truth yet, like Bunyan's pilgrim, we have soldiered on. We have become the present-day pilgrims, going on marches and attending rallies and events where we can hear the truth from those brave enough to speak out, and who have risked being ostracised and often lost their jobs as a result.

Here is the second verse:

Whoso beset him round
With dismal stories.
Do but themselves confound,
His strength the more is.
No lion can him fright
He'll with a giant fight,
But he will have the right
To be a pilgrim.

We know only too well who beset us round with dismal stories – the World Economic Forum, the World Health Organisation, the Bill and Melinda Gates Foundation, the government, the media, the drug companies and the climate change activists. And yes, they do themselves confound as, with every pronouncement the mainstream makes, we grow stronger. True, we are fighting with giants, with rich and mighty organisations, but who won the fight between David and Goliath in the end? The dismal stories that have surfaced recently warn of a new and even more dangerous Covid strain now going round but we, the pilgrims, know to take no notice.

Here is the third and final verse:

> *Hobgoblin nor foul fiend*
> *Can daunt his spirit.*
> *He knows he at the end*
> *Shall life inherit.*
> *Then fancies flee away*
> *He'll fear not what men say.*
> *He'll labour night and day*
> *To be a pilgrim.*

The hobgoblins and foul fiends of today are the politicians, health secretaries, chief medical officers, pharmaceutical giants, university modellers and so on, who have done their level best to daunt our spirits but they have not succeeded. We have feared not what men say, although sometimes it has been very hard to withstand the abuse, name-calling and accusations of being Covid and climate change deniers and conspiracy theorists, and we still have a fight on. Only last week Alice Thomson was writing in the *Times* that our best defences against the new variant are the boosters and flu jabs. This is in face of overwhelming evidence that the mRNA jabs are not only completely ineffective against the virus but have caused untold damage and even death to many people.

In the *Daily Mail* on Thursday, former Woman's Hour presenter Jenni Murray wrote that she had been taken to hospital on New Year's Eve with double pneumonia and that she needed oxygen. She added: 'For goodness sake, I was jabbed beyond reason. I'd had the Covid vaccine, the flu jab and a pneumonia jab that I thought would protect me.'

The other day, my next door neighbour told me that another neighbour had gone down with Covid. When I said, 'With all the jabs she's had I'm not surprised,' he gave an exasperated sigh and said, 'There you go again.' Such stories remind us that we pilgrims have a long way to go before the penny finally drops – that the jabs CAUSE illness, not prevent it. All too many people are still not listening.

Yes, we do have to labour night and day, never letting up, but my hope is that even if we don't inherit life ourselves, or the life that we would like, that at least we are trying to make the world a better place for our children and grandchildren by being brave enough to stand fearlessly for the right, whatever the cost.

So thank you, John Bunyan, for composing that hymn all those years ago. We should remind ourselves that he wrote it in prison while serving a 12-year sentence for preaching without a licence. His captivity gave him the strength and courage to write a book and a hymn that is read and sung to this day. Perhaps we should take heed of his words as never before.

New friendships form

THERE IS AN OLD SAYING: it's an ill wind that blows nobody any good. The truth of this has come home to me recently, as, although the past few years have been horrendous thanks to the Covid and allied hysteria, there have also been some surprising and unlooked-for benefits.

Chief of these has been the forming of new friendships among the enlightened and the awakened.

Just before Christmas, I found a bottle of champagne outside my door with a note saying, "You and *The Conservative Woman* have kept me sane over the past four years.' I had no idea who this mysterious benefactor might be, as the note was signed with a name I did not recognise. There was, however, on the note an Oxford address.

I did wonder how this person discovered my address and got into the building to deliver the bubbly, but I sent him a note of thanks and included my email and phone number in case he wanted to make further contact. The upshot was that we met for coffee and instantly became firm friends. Although we met as complete strangers, we chatted for hours and it was as if we had known each other all our lives. We have arranged to meet again for further discussions as it is so wonderful to find an ally, especially in Oxford where the majority still seem to adhere to the mainstream narrative.

My new Oxford friend – a gay man in his mid-50s – bemoaned the fact that he can no longer have any proper exchanges with his former friends, including other gay men. He thought the reason for this was that many gays have felt ostracised for so many years that all they want to do now is to belong, rather than risking being outsiders once more by questioning the official line.

It is even true that in many cases, thanks to the way society has divided over Covid, one cannot now have a proper relationship with one's own family. My new friend's sister has had all the jabs and as a probable results now suffers from an auto-immune disease. But she continues to believe that the vaccine is safe and effective and reckons her once sensible brother has gone mad.

Another friend has joined a local group who are all 'one of us'. She says it is such a comfort to go along to meetings as her own family believe she is crazy for being vehemently anti-vax (anti Covid vax at least) and a climate change denier. Her family, she says, simply don't want to listen to what she has to say, never mind that she has done all the research and they haven't. They 'follow the science' whereas she questions it. She asks: why am I so different from every other member of my family?

It is something I have also often asked myself while shaking my head at the rubbish so many supposedly intelligent people are prepared to take on board.

For my friend, her neighbourhood group has become her new family.

Last year I was doing a photoshoot for a newspaper and the photographer warned me about the make-up artist who had come to make me camera-ready (or as near as I am likely to get). 'She's completely off the wall,' the photographer said. 'She's anti-vax, anti-lockdown and anti all the Covid policies.' Great, I thought, she's one of us – and once again, we had a long discussion as we compared notes and discovered that we thought alike on all these issues.

We Covid sceptics have formed a merry band and although we discuss very serious matters, we can laugh and joke together as well, especially at all the nonsense that has been pushed at us over the last four years.

But what I've realised, sometimes painfully, is that when it comes to 'them' and 'us', there is no way of telling in advance into which camp one's friends, family and colleagues might fall. The only explanation I can offer is that some of us hear the click, and others just don't. It's a bit like having perfect pitch. Some people can sing beautifully in tune and accurately reproduce notes they hear on a piano, for instance. Others can't and their ears will never be attuned. Or maybe it's a bit like having a gift for languages. I have friends who pick up new languages very easily and others who can't speak in a foreign tongue even when they have lived in the host country for years.

So I think that the ability to see through to the truth has to be a kind of gift, because one thing I have learned through all this is that you cannot persuade those who firmly adhere to 'the science' and the mainstream narrative to change their views. There is no point in telling them to stop testing themselves with the PCR kit as they simply take no notice. We can only hope that as time goes on, ever more people will hear the click and adjust their former beliefs accordingly. I like to think that we are winning, although it is proving a long hard struggle.

Meanwhile, I am very grateful for the new friends and allies I have made through all this as they give me great solace and help me to understand that I am not so much out on a limb as I once imagined.

JANUARY 29, 2024

Breathtaking indeed

AFTER THE ALMOST UNIVERSALLY ADULATORY reviews from TV critics for the 'gritty' and 'harrowing' hospital drama *Breathtaking*, about the first six months of the Covid outbreak, plus an admonition from the Evening Standard that it should be made compulsory viewing, comes a refreshing corrective from *Daily Mail* writer Andrew Pierce.

The headline said: 'How the holier-than-thou doctor behind ITV's new Covid drama is a Tory-hating activist who doesn't always get her facts right.' The article went on to enumerate the 'facts' that writer and doctor Rachel Clarke, on whose 2021 memoir the series was based, doesn't always get right.

For those who had not heard of 52-year-old Dr Clarke before this three-part drama series aired, including me, here are a few biographical details. Whether or not they are 'facts' may be open to question. She says she comes from a family of doctors and read PPE (Philosophy, Politics and Economics) at Oxford. After that she became a high-profile TV documentary maker but gave it all up to take science A-levels in her late 20s to gain entry to medical school. In 2003, at the age of 29, she started studying for a medical degree at University College, London, transferring to Oxford two years later to complete her studies. She qualified as a doctor in 2009. Dr Clarke was a driving force behind the junior doctors' strike in 2016 and has in recent years specialised in palliative care.

A few Google searches reveal that she is a vocal left-wing activist who during the early days of Covid was a ferocious campaigner for harder, stricter lockdowns and compulsory mask-wearing. This drew an anguished response from *Telegraph* cartoonist Bob Moran, whose severely disabled eight-year-old daughter nearly died from being deprived of medical care during lockdown and could not understand why people were wearing masks and distancing themselves from her.

He wrote an angry, if ill-advised tweet in September 2021 saying that Dr Clarke should be 'verbally abused' for the harm she has caused. Dr Clarke was quick to reply with her own tweet: 'Why do you employ a man who openly abuses NHS staff, *Telegraph?*' She reported Bob to the police and the *Telegraph* sacked him, even though he apologised to Dr Clarke. While admitting that his tweet was out of order, Bob said that lockdown and other measures implemented to try and control a virus which poses no threat to children, have been devastating.

As regards Rachel Clarke, as well as being a caring doctor, she is also a prolific writer and TV personality. Thanks perhaps to her dual talents, interviewers in every branch of the media have accorded her the kind of reverential attention usually reserved for royalty and world spiritual leaders. She was described by the *Guardian* as 'one of the best doctor writers to emerge within a rich new scene.' Because, as well as working with patients who have very, very grave and serious things wrong with them (her words), Dr Clarke writes regularly for the *Guardian, New York*

Times, *New Statesman* and *BMJ* as well as frequently appearing on TV and radio. She has also written three books billed as *Sunday Times* bestsellers, with a fourth due out later this year. One wonders where she finds the time to attend to her gravely ill patients.

So what about the facts that are 'not quite right'? Doubts were first raised on her claimed credentials by Miriam Finch, who writes a Substack called *Informed Consent Matters*, under the name Miri AF. In an open letter to various health professionals, Miri points out anomalies in the TV doctor's apparent qualifications. It is not possible, she says, to transfer to Oxford after two years at another medical college, as Oxford does not accept such students. You would have to start from scratch, and this would mean that Dr Clarke qualified in 2011, not 2009. Miri adds, though, that it is well-nigh impossible for lay people to verify academic claims made by doctors. It is also possible, of course, that an exception was made in her case, as a mature student.

However, this is one aspect which has been taken up by a number of people including James Delingpole, who asked: 'Who is she?' Dr Clarke replied in one of her endless tweets, 'Who am I, James? It's such a tantalising question. If only there were written sources that could shed light on the sinister mystery.' Dr Clarke is not above sarcastic putdowns, then. Many of her 217,000 adoring followers rubbished Delingpole as a 'nobody' while praising Dr Clarke to the skies following this exchange.

The *Mail*'s Andrew Pierce queries other claims made by Dr Clarke. In a recent Guardian interview with Zoe Williams, Dr Clarke said she was 'the first medical student to have a baby while studying at Oxford.' Now I know for a fact that this is not true as my university flatmate, also a medical student, had a baby while studying for her degree. Then a *Daily Mail* reader wrote in to say that female medical students at his university 50 years ago were regularly giving birth while studying, and nobody thought this was anything odd.

But, Pierce adds: 'A fondness for hyperbole is typical of Clarke's decidedly partisan worldwiew.'

During the recent doctors' strikes, Dr Clarke repeatedly stated that a junior doctor's starting pay is £14.09 per hour, about the same a shelf-filler at a supermarket. Yet Full Fact has roundly dismissed this figure, pointing out that even the lowest-ranked junior doctors earn more than this.

When it came to Brexit, she called for a second referendum, maintaining that one-third of NHS beds at her hospitals had been closed due to our exit from the EU. Yet this remark was made before Britain had actually left. She also stated, in a 2018 interview with Victoria Derbyshire, that a third of in-patient beds had to be closed because 'some of our very best European nurses from Italy, Portugal, Spain, have already gone back home because they have been made to feel so unwelcome and so unwanted post-Brexit.' This was not matched, Pierce points out, 'by any meaningful results.'

Dr Clarke has stated that she began working in palliative care, firstly at the John Radcliffe Hospital in Oxford and later the Horton General Hospital in Banbury. But she is not registered at either of these hospitals, and the Katharine House Hospice in Oxfordshire, where she supposedly also worked, refused to confirm this to Pierce with the remark, 'We can't say anything about that.' According to the *Daily Mail* preview of the series on Monday February 19th, Dr Clarke was working in a big city hospital during the early days of the pandemic.

Er ... Which big city hospital, exactly?

More recently, when Sir Keir Starmer falsely accused Prime Minister Rishi Sunak of making transphobic jokes in the Commons, Dr Clarke wrote: 'To make transphobic jokes in Parliament is bad enough. To make them in front of the grieving mother of a child murdered in a transphobic attack is absolutely reprehensible. Shame on Sunak.' The fact that Esther Ghey, the mother of the murdered teenager Brianna Ghey, was not in the House at the time, was a minor detail. But never let the facts ..

The TV drama certainly laid it on thick. The heroic female doctor played by Joanne Froggatt, wore not only a mask but a visor as well as a stethoscope, reminiscent of the 1950s Doctor films starring Dirk Bogarde. When she removed the mask, her face was disfigured with mask lines. The make-up department certainly went to town, making her look haggard and with stringy unwashed hair to complete the image of the saintly medic working under almost impossible conditions to the detriment of her wellbeing and her own family.

But was the series, intended to tug at our heartstrings, accurate? Many doctors and nurses working in hospitals during the early days of Covid say no, that it was, rather, a shameless piece of propaganda and only marginally based on what was happening. The supposed overwhelming of NHS hospitals and services was, they say, vastly exaggerated.

For *Times* TV critic Hugo Rifkind, though, writing under the headline 'Take your medicine – watch this Covid drama' it 'oozed bleak authenticity' and the real villains all along were the Covid deniers.

Does he mean those of us who have doggedly tried to get at the truth, rather than supinely believing every word of an overheated television drama and a publicity-hungry doctor? He surely does, as the late Derek Jameson used to say on his amusing 1984 TV series about how foreign television stations depicted the British.

Why not celebrate wellness for a change?

IF NOTHING ELSE, THE EVENTS of the past four years have focused attention on illness as never before. Week after week, radio and television stations and print media run stories about how celebrities and others have faced life-threatening illnesses and conditions and bravely fought through.

For instance, in last week's *Times Magazine*, there were no fewer than three big stories about serious illness. The first was an interview with the new *Today* presenter Emma Barnett, whisked away from *Woman's Hour*, about her endometriosis and struggle with IVF. She was featured on the cover, looking as sultry and glamorous as ever and billed as talking about 'her private trauma.'

Yes, so private that it was splashed all over the pages of a major magazine. And it's not the first time, by a long way, that Emma Barnett has spoken or written about her health and fertility issues.

In the same issue of the magazine, former broadcaster Alastair Stewart – also featured on the cover – talks about the day he was told he had dementia. Further on in the magazine, foreign correspondent Sebastian Junger is interviewed about his biggest battle for survival, when an artery ruptured in his abdomen and he nearly bled to death.

It seems that we have a ghoulish fascination with illness that is growing all the time. The so-called Good Health pages of newspapers are always about illness, and every day some new celebrity comes forward with their cancer, arthritis, depression, diabetes, autism, menopause, ME or other 'journey'. Then, as often as not, they make television shows about the battle with their condition, whatever that may be.

There are also endless books and memoirs pouring out about the authors' problems with severe, lifelong illness. We can expect a slew of material about 'my battle with long Covid'. Some have been published already. Sometimes the authors are famous, sometimes not. Sometimes they are made famous purely because of their illness. It seems that publishers love nothing more than a harrowing account of living with chronic illness.

But why not celebrate wellness for a change? I wrote an article in the current issue of *The Oldie* magazine, saying that at the age of 80 I have never been ill in my life. The editor Harry Mount (cheeky boy!) labelled me 'Superwoman'. He believes that there are many oldies who, like me, are completely fit and well, but that we are never mentioned. Instead, the emphasis, especially as we get older, is on all the ills that flesh is heir to.

Well, I'm not particularly a superwoman. I just don't go around looking for illnesses and am certainly not going to be dragooned into queueing up for the latest jabs and boosters. As I point out in the article, my lasting good health – so far at least – has nothing to do with the ministrations of the medical profession.

My ex-husband Neville, a former medical correspondent and frequent contributor to *The Conservative Woman*, is also perfectly well and says he has not been to a doctor for over 50 years.

The other week, an 86-year-old friend from childhood was staying with me, as I am writing his life story. He read my *Oldie* article and told me that he, too, was as fit as a fiddle. He goes skiing, plays golf, swims every day, is still working and says he is about to take up tennis again. As a young man, he was a county champion. He told me he was fed up with reading all the illness stories in the newspapers and longed for some positive, upbeat and happy tales instead. He added that at this stage of his life he didn't want to be made miserable all the time or labelled decrepit because of his age.

Over the years, there have been several attempts to launch publications that concentrate on good or happy news, and none has succeeded. We are told that positive stories 'write white'; in other words, they are not compelling or dramatic enough to engage the reader, and this is why in recent years misery memoirs, of which Charles Spencer's about his brutal boarding school days, is the latest, have become bestsellers.

But is this always true? Jane Austen said, 'let other pens dwell on guilt and misery' and her novels are still enjoyed the world over, and frequently dramatized for the screen. Jilly Cooper's jolly upbeat stories have been wildly popular, although she does introduce a darker note in her latest, *Tackle!*, when Taggie, the wife of her hero Rupert Campbell-Black, has recently had a cancer diagnosis. Was she required by the publishers to put that in, one wonders, to make the book seem more modern and relevant?

I also believe that the rags-to-riches story of my friend, who left school at 14 with no qualifications to work as a builder's labourer and ended up in the *Sunday Times* Rich List, is at least as gripping as any tale of sadness, serious illness and loss.

While so many friends and neighbours, including some members of my own family, have gone down with Covid, or what passes for it, I have not had so much as a sniffle, no thanks to testing, jabs, masks, lockdowns or any of the other nonsense thrown at us. And at my age I am supposed to be 'vulnerable.' I'm sure I would have been a gibbering wreck by now if I had obeyed any of the strictures, instead of the hundred per cent healthy octogenarian I actually am.

We've experienced so much doom and gloom over the past four years, much of it fabricated, that surely we now need some serious cheering up. So let us commend the well, the successful, the brave, the happy and those who have risen above all the propaganda and fearmongering to remain in fine fettle, rather than constantly dwelling on sickness and disease.

The final entry – hot on the heels of Dr Rachel Clarke, here comes – Dr Michael Mosley

ON FRIDAY JULY 12, the BBC is to devote a whole day's programming to honour the late Dr Michael Mosley, the popular media doctor who advised us to fast two days a week, stand on one leg, have cold showers and spend hours every day doing squats and sit-ups. Announcing the 'Just One Thing Day', Radio 4 controller Mohit Bakaya said: 'Michael's broadcasting changed people's lives, so we thought it would be fitting to dedicate a day to the impact he had and celebrate his legacy within broadcasting and beyond.'

Michael Mosley came across as a cheery chappie, who dispensed apparent medical and scientific advice as if from a great height, and his affable demeanour seemed to give weight to all his confident pronouncements.

But – what exactly was his legacy? Apart from the diet books which popularised intermittent fasting, Mosley was a vociferous and relentless public pusher of the Covid vaccines. And strangely enough, since his death last month, among all the fulsome tributes there was no mention of this indefatigable, never-ending plugging.

So here I am to fill you in where the BBC will not.

Starting in May 2020, Mosley published a 'popular' book, *Covid-19: Everything you need to know about the Coronavirus and the race for the vaccine.* The publisher's blurb read: 'From award-winning science journalist Dr Michael Mosley: the story of Covid-19 – the greatest public health threat of our time.' A 'safe and effective' vaccine, according to Mosley, was the 'only way to beat the virus.'

That was the first blast but by no means the last. On March 12, 2021 he wrote in the *Daily Mail:* 'I recently got a Covid jab – AstraZeneca as it happens. It was all incredibly easy and apart from the brief sting of the injection I had no side effect – except cockiness.'

He went on in that article to address the alleged downsides of the vaccine, such as that it alters your DNA, makes you sterile, actually gives you Covid and that the shots were not to be trusted as they had been developed too quickly. Perhaps needless to say he dismissed them all as so much myth and nonsense, at the same time advising readers to get a second jab to make sure they were well and truly protected.

Although Mosley carefully nurtured his reputation for being smiley and affable, this was only a front. He wrote: 'I told an unvaccinated friend that I didn't want her to come to a social gathering because of the risk she posed' and he castigated Dr Steve James for objecting to mandatory jabs for NHS workers. Mosley concluded this article by saying, 'I'm convinced we have Covid on the run, once vaccine-hesitant people will realise the benefits of being jabbed. The race to develop a vaccine has been truly extraordinary.'

One January 14, 2022 he announced in his *Daily Mail* column that the vaccine programme had saved more than 100,000 lives and prevented others from ending up in hospital and suffering from long Covid. Reflecting on the fact that five million people in the UK had chosen not to be vaccinated, he said wearily that these people seem to think they are not at risk or that natural immunity will save them. It won't, he argued. He informed us that the unvaccinated and unboosted made up the majority of those currently in intensive care and assured readers that a course of vaccines conferred 75 per cent protection against the virus. He hammered this home by adding that having a second or third jab amplifies and refines your immune system.

But, oh dear! In spite of having every jab going and boasting that the only side-effect he suffered from was cockiness, he announced on May 20, 2022 that he had gone down with a bout of Covid himself. He wrote: 'After more than two years dodging the Covid-19 bullet, I have been struck down. This is particularly galling because throughout the pandemic I've tried to reduce my risk by avoiding packed places, such as pubs, and wearing a mask on public transport and in shops.'

In typical jaunty style, Mosley gave his tips for dealing with this nasty virus, such as taking exercise, keeping hydrated, resting and even singing in the shower. And here, once again, was a chance to promote a vaccine; a nasal one this time, as the virus, he told us, enters through the nose. He also stated that Omicron was the fastest-spreading virus in human history but that those who were fully vaccinated were 85 per cent less likely to die from this strain than the unvaccinated.

Omicron? Whatever happened to it? It vanished without trace and we haven't heard about it for at least a couple of years. And did anybody ever die from Omicron, vaccinated or not?

Michael Mosley himself died without ever raising any doubts, at least publicly, about the efficacy of the mRNA vaccines. *Au contraire*, he wrote about them as if they were the most wonderful invention of all time. Although his programmes, articles and podcasts were said to be 'utterly rooted in science' he conveniently ignored all the growing evidence from scientists and doctors who were casting doubt on the safety and efficacy of the vaccines, and never once referred to their findings.

We now know that several TV doctors who promoted the jab were paid by vaccine companies, sometimes in quite large sums. It has not been revealed whether Mosley was among them but was he even an actual doctor?

Well, yes and no. He graduated from Oxford University with a degree in PPE, rather like Rachel Clarke, mentioned earlier. This course often leads to a high-profile career in politics but on graduation Mosley went into banking. After a few years, again much like Rachel Clarke, he jacked it in to train as a doctor. This was at the Royal Free Hospital Medical School in London, a course which lasts at least five years. But – and this is the crucial point – *'Doctor' Mosley never practised as a doctor, not even for one minute.*

Instead, he went straight onto an Assistant Producer's course at the BBC where his easy and pleasant television manner soon ensured he became a broadcasting star. He was, perhaps, somewhat more of a real doctor than First Lady 'Dr' Jill Biden, but not much, and nor was he a scientist.

His 5:2 diet, written with Mimi Spencer, although the lion's share of the credit went to Mosley, may have helped those who were able to follow it, but I hope that history will show that under the cheery chappie upbeat carapace, Mosley was a dangerously deluded and deeply sinister man who never stopped beating the drum for what is fast emerging as one of the most harmful and destructive medical interventions of modern times and possibly, of all time.

That's some legacy!

_____

Michael Mosley died on or around June 5, 2024, aged 67, while going for a walk in intense heat on the Greek island of Symi. His death was recorded as 'natural causes' but mystery surrounds his demise such as, why did he go for a walk without his phone, in midday, and why, in spite of intense searching by police, drones, helicopters and volunteers, was his body not found for five days? It seems we may never know the answers.

This article above was among the most read of my pieces, or indeed any piece, on The Conservative Woman website and showed that many people were not fooled by Mosley's confident pronouncements about the Covid vaccines.

This seems to be a fitting place to conclude my Covid Diary but the story is far from over. We can only hope that as time goes on, the truth will overturn the lies, falsehoods and propaganda we have been fed since Covid-19 was first announced as being the most dread disease in human history.

_____

Acknowledgements

I AM ETERNALLY GRATEFUL TO Kathy Gyngell, Margaret Ashworth, Alan Ashworth and the rest of the team at *The Conservative Woman*, now named *TCW Defending Freedom*, for publishing my articles and for alerting people generally to the great harms that were done to the whole world by implementation of the Covid policies.

Glossary

ALTHOUGH THIS IS NOT A technical publication, a few simple explanations of medical and scientific terms mentioned in the Diary, and much bandied about during Covid, might be in order. They have been kindly provided by my ex-husband Neville Hodgkinson, former medical and science correspondent at *The Sunday Times*, and frequent contributor to *TCW*.

What are PCR tests?

PCR stands for polymerase chain reaction, a process that looks for a stretch of DNA in a biological sample and multiplies it many times to make it easily accessible. Kary Mullis, the American scientist who won the Nobel prize in chemistry for inventing it, urged caution in its use as a diagnostic tool but it was misused in exactly that way during the Covid scare, leading to many false positive results. Finding a trace of viral DNA and multiplying it up with the PCR test does not mean there is necessarily active infection, with risk of illness or risk of passing on an infection to others.

What is a lateral flow test?

This is a device that detects the presence of a specific molecule in a biological sample without the need for specialized equipment. In the Covid test, the target molecule is a molecular structure from the virus's surface called an antigen. It gets that name because when recognized by the immune system, antibodies are created that help to block its spread in the body. The test kit contains antibodies which react with virus antigen when there is active infection in the sample being tested. These kits are a generally reliable tool in tracking disease spread, with a false positive rate claimed to be only 0.3 per cent. However, using them to test millions of healthy children still meant there were thousands of false alarms, and unnecessary classroom closures.

What are mRNA vaccines?

The letters stand for Messenger RiboNucleic Acid. The vaccines were designed to induce our bodies to make a specific protein, the toxic 'spike' of the genetically engineered Covid virus, in the hope that this would increase our immunity to the virus. It was originally claimed that the genetic material would act only at the site of the injection, and that it would soon disappear. Both claims have been disproved, with studies showing that the nanoparticles carrying the genetic instruction for 'spike' travel all over the body and can be long-lasting.

Meanwhile, the Covid saga rumbles on, with supposedly new variants, such as FLIRT being discovered, causing an apparent rise in cases. We are still being urged to test ourselves regularly, and mask mandates are being reimposed in many medical settings. We must fight this for all we are worth.

Select Bibliography

Bell, Rudolph M: Holy Anorexia. University of Chicago Press, 1987

Hodgkinson, Neville: How HIV/Aids set the stage for the Covid crisis. UK Book Publishing, 2022

Jones, Alex: The Great Reset and the War for the World. Skyhorse, 2022

Jupp, Daniel: Gates of Hell: Why Bill Gates is the most dangerous man in the world. Bombardier Books, 2023

Kennedy, Robert F. Jr: The Real Anthony Fauci, Bill Gates, Pharma and the Global War on Democracy and Public Health. Children's Health Defense, 2022.